Clinical Methods in
Obstetrics and Gynecology
A problem based approach

Clinical Methods in Obstetrics and Gynecology
A problem based approach

Second edition

EDITOR
ASHA OUMACHIGUI
MD
Formerly Director-Professor and Head
Department of Obstetrics and Gynecology
Jawaharlal Institute of Postgraduate Medical Education and Research, Pondicherry

CO-EDITORS
S. SOUNDARA RAGHAVAN
MD DGO
Professor
Department of Obstetrics and Gynecology
Jawaharlal Institute of Postgraduate Medical Education and Research, Pondicherry

S. HABEEBULLAH
MD MNAMS
Director-Professor and Head
Department of Obstetrics and Gynecology
Jawaharlal Institute of Postgraduate Medical Education and Research, Pondicherry

FOREWORD
S. N. MUKHERJEE

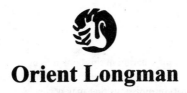

Orient Longman

Dedicated to our parents and our teachers

Orient Longman Private Limited

Registered Office
3-6-272 Himayatnagar, Hyderabad 500 019 (AP) India
cogeneral@orientlongman.com

Other offices
Bangalore/Bhopal/Bhubaneshwar/Chandigarh/
Chennai/Ernakulam/Guwahati/Hyderabad/Jaipur/
Kolkata/Lucknow/Mumbai/New Delhi/Patna

Typeset by
Trinity Designers & Typesetters
Chennai 600 041

Printed in India by offset at
SS Colour Impression Pvt Ltd
Chennai 600 106

Published by
Orient Longman Private Limited
160 Anna Salai
Chennai 600 002
chegeneral@orientlongman.com

ISBN 13: 978-81-250-3078-2
ISBN 10: 81-250-3078-6

Foreword

This innovative book *Clinical Methods in Obstetrics and Gynecology: A problem based approach* is a welcome addition to the field of obstetrics and gynecology. An Indian textbook on a clinical approach to the subject was long overdue. This important publication is timely and meets the needs of students and practising physicians. It is a sincere effort to initiate students to learn obstetrics and gynecology in the proper perspective.

It is sad to see that many of the younger physicians lack adequate clinical skills to solve the patient's problems; students too, generally do not acquire the necessary skills during their clinical postings. The contibutors to this volume have focused as much on the subject as on the central theme of learning clinical skills. The book is edited by three eminent teachers in obstetrics and gynecology of Jawaharlal Institute of Postgraduate Medical Education and Research (JIPMER), Pondicherry. The faculty members of this esteemed institution have worked towards a competency-based curriculum for many years. The institution is well known for bringing about innovations in medical education. Indeed the book makes a valuable contribution towards highlighting both the critical needs of clinical skills development and necessary strategies for providing quality reproductive health services.

The first chapter on communication with the patient, and history-taking emphasises the importance of interpersonal communication skills and the need to create and maintain a sound doctor–patient relationship. The scientific content of the book is of a high calibre. The book contains important topics of current interest and provides valuable information. The chapters are comprehensive, educative and up-to-date. The volume is superbly crafted to prove user-friendly. The editors must be complimented for their excellent work. It is fervently hoped that this brilliant publication will be widely used by students and physicians practising obstetrics and gynecology.

Professor S. N. Mukherjee
Formerly Professor and Head
Department of Obstetrics and Gynecology
HP Medical College, Simla
JIPMER, Pondicherry
Maulana Azad Medical College & LNJP Hospital, New Delhi
University College of Medical Sciences & Safdarjung Hospital, New Delhi

*A man would do nothing, if he waited until he could do it so well
that no one would find fault with what he has done.*

Cardinal Newman

Preface to the second edition

We are happy that this book has gone into the second edition and we write this preface with great pleasure. As in the first edition, we seek to re-emphasise that students must acquire the skills of gathering information through history taking and physical examination, and learn the art and science of interpreting data and selecting relevant investigations. The delivery pattern of health care, especially for women, needs to be woman-centered rather than technology driven.

The first edition was well received by those who saw the book. The necessity of a book on clinical methods in the specialty of obstetrics and gynecology is absolute, especially in India where we can ill afford to rely on technology alone. We hope that this book will ultimately help budding doctors to appreciate and value the clinical approach.

In bringing out this edition, we were encouraged by the comments of our esteemed colleagues. We have taken into account their feedback and have added two chapters: antenatal care and hypertensive disorders in pregnancy. All the illustrations have also been redrawn. It was tempting to add more information, but that would have detracted from the primary intent of this book: to give only as much information as is required for interpretation of symptoms and signs; readers are requested to consult standard textbooks for details.

We are grateful to our publishers for bringing out the second edition and to Mr Rangarajan for drawing the illustrations accurately. Our special thanks to the cover designer Mr Bhanu Bhasker.

Asha Oumachigui
S. Soundara Raghavan
S. Habeebullah

Preface to the first edition

This book has been written for undergraduate and postgraduate students, to enable them to learn clinical skills necessary to solve problems with which their patients present. Students must acquire the art of gathering useful information from history-taking, physical examination and relevant investigations. Increasingly, expensive investigations are replacing history-taking and physical examination. These investigations are certainly beneficial to the patient, if they are employed in the context of clinical findings/diagnosis, but may often be unaffordable in developing countries. They must be used for patient care intelligently, economically, and above all, with compassion.

There is currently a growing concern that a good number of doctors do not possess adequate clinical skills. The Ninth Five Year Plan Document on Health notes: 'One of the important reasons for suboptimal performance of healthcare institutions is the poor quality and inappropriateness of education and training of healthcare providers, resulting in a lack of problem-solving competencies and skills.' This has significant relevance in the light of the country's commitment to the implementation of reproductive and child health (RCH) programmes.

The faculty members at the Jawaharlal Institute of Postgraduate Medical Education and Research, Pondicherry, during the last 15 years, have worked towards a competency-based curriculum. Evaluation has shown that 80 to 90 per cent of students who have followed this curriculum are well versed with essential skills required for rendering RCH care. Besides having experience in training undergraduates and postgraduates, the faculty members have also brought about innovations in medical education.

This book may be used to guide undergraduate students as they begin their posting in obstetrics and gynecology. The aim is to help students acquire skills of communication, history-taking and physical examination. They must also be proficient in taking decisions with regard to selection of investigations, choosing appropriate options for treatment, while keeping in mind the patient's background.

The knowledge provided in this book is only to explain why a specific piece of information is sought from history or physical findings, or to justify the selection of an investigation. Therefore, students should refer to standard textbooks in order to gain indepth information. References are provided at the end of the book.

The first three chapters deal with communication and history-taking, general examination and gynecologic and obstetric examination. In the rest of the chapters, approach to common problems in obstetrics, neonatology and gynecology is discussed. The list of problems was consolidated after consulting colleagues from different parts of the country, so as to ensure relevance. It was considered necessary to include the chapter *Strategies for skill learning* as this specialty is predominantly skill-based. Trainee teachers would find this chapter useful. A list of learning objectives given at the beginning of each chapter is meant to promote self-learning. A clinical scenario is presented to start the discussion and to make learning clinically oriented. 'Knowledge is treasure but practice is its key' goes a Chinese proverb. We hope that this book will be a step towards bridging the gap between theory and practice when training students.

Asha Oumachigui
S. Soundara Raghavan
S. Habeebullah

Acknowledgement

We appreciate the help rendered by our colleagues in JIPMER:
1. Dr. Lalita Kulkarni, MBBS, MS
    Former Senior Resident, Dept. of Anatomy
2. Dr. Latha Chaturvedula, MD, DNB
    Associate Professor, Dept. of Obstetrics and Gynecology
3. Dr. S. Srividya, MD, DNB
    Former Senior Resident, Dept. of Obstetrics and Gynecology
4. Dr. J. L. Baidya, MD
    Former Senior Resident, Dept. of Obstetrics and Gynecology
5. Mrs. D. Kalaichelvi and Mr. B. Pandiadurai for secretarial assistance

Contributors

1. **Aparna Agrawal,** MD
   Associate Professor,
   Dept. of Medicine, JIPMER

2. **N. Ananthakrishnan,** MS, FRCS, FAMS
   Director-Professor and Head,
   Dept. of Surgery, JIPMER
   Faculty Member, National Teacher Training Centre, JIPMER, Pondicherry

3. **B. Vishnu Bhat,** MD, DHA, DDE
   Professor,
   Dept. of Pediatrics (Neonatology), JIPMER
   Faculty Member, National Teacher Training Centre, JIPMER, Pondicherry

4. **A. Bupathy,** MD, DGO
   Professor,
   Dept. of Obstetrics and Gynecology, JIPMER

5. **R. Chandrasekaran,** MD
   Professor and Head,
   Dept. of Psychiatry, JIPMER

6. **S. Habeebullah,** MD, MNAMS
   Director-Professor and Head,
   Dept. of Obstetrics and Gynecology, JIPMER

7. **Asha Oumachigui,** MD
   Former Director-Professor and Head,
   Dept. of Obstetrics and Gynecology, JIPMER
   Faculty Member, National Teacher Training Centre, JIPMER, Pondicherry

8. **Gita Rajagopalan,** MD, DGO
   Professor,
   Dept. of Obstetrics and Gynecology, JIPMER

9. **P. Reddi Rani,** MD, DGO
    Professor,
    Dept. of Obstetrics and Gynecology, JIPMER

10. **Rajeev Singh,** MD, DNB
    Former Senior Resident,
    Dept. of Obstetrics and Gynecology, JIPMER

11. **S. Soundara Raghavan,** MD, DGO
    Professor,
    Dept. of Obstetrics and Gynecology, JIPMER

Abbreviations

ACA	anticardiolipin antibody	CT	clotting time
ACE	angiotensin converting enzyme	D and C	dilatation and curettage
ARDS	adult respiratory distress syndrome	DFMC	daily fetal movement count
		DES	diethyl stilbesterol
AFLP	acute fatty liver of pregnancy	DIC	disseminated intravascular coagulation
ALT	alanine aminotransferase		
ANC	antenatal care	DMPA	depot medroxy progesterone acetate
Anti-HBc (IgM)	anti-hepatitis B core immunoglobulin M	DNA	deoxyribonucleic acid
APH	antepartum hemorrhage	DUB	dysfunctional uterine bleeding
APTT	activated partial thromboplastin time	ECG	electrocardiogram
		EDD	expected date of delivery
ARM	artificial rupture of membranes	EEG	electroencephalogram
ART	assisted reproductive techniques	ESR	erythrocyte sedimentation rate
		FDP	fibrin degradation products
AST	aspartate aminotransferase	FNAC	fine needle aspiration cytology
BD	twice daily	FSH	follicle stimulating hormone
BFP-ST	biological false positive test for syphilis	GnRH	gonadotrophin releasing hormone
BMI	body mass index	GTT	glucose tolerance test
BP	blood pressure	HAV	hepatitis A virus
CAT	computerised axial tomography	Hb	hemoglobin
		HBeAg	hepatitis B envelope antigen
CCF	congestive cardiac failure	HBsAg	hepatitis B surface antigen
CLASP	collaborative low dose aspirin in pregnancy	hCG	human chorionic gonadotrophin
CNS	central nervous system	HCV	hepatitis C virus
COC	combination oral contraceptive	HELLP	hemolysis, elevated liver enzymes, low platelet
CPD	cephalopelvic disproportion		
CRP	C-reactive protein	HEV	hepatitis E virus

HIV	human immunodeficiency virus	P/V	per vaginum
HLA	human lymphocyte antigen	Pap smear	Papanicolaou smear
HMD	hyaline membrane disease	PCOS	polycystic ovarian syndrome
HRT	hormone replacement therapy	PCT	progesterone challenge test
IgG	immunoglobulin G	PGE_2	prostaglandin E_2
IgM	immunoglobulin M	PGF_2	prostaglandin F_2
IHCP	intrahepatic cholestasis of pregnancy	PID	pelvic inflammatory disease
IM	intramuscular	PIH	pregnancy induced hypertension
IUCD	intrauterine contraceptive device	POG	period of gestation
IUD	intrauterine death	PPH	postpartum hemorrhage
IUGR	intrauterine growth restriction	PROM	premature rupture of membrane
IV	intravenous	PTT	partial thromboplastin time
KCT	kaolin clotting time	QID	four times daily
KOH	potassium hydroxide	RFT	renal function test
LA	lupus anticoagulant	RPL	recurrent pregnancy loss
LBW	low birth weight	RTI	reproductive tract infection
LDH	lactic dehydrogenase	SC	subcutaneous
LFT	liver function test	SLE	systemic lupus erythematosus
LH	luteinising hormone	SFH	symphysiofundal height
LMP	last menstrual period	SSRI	serotonin specific reuptake inhibitors
LPD	luteal phase defects	STD	sexually transmitted diseases
$MgSO_4$	magnesium sulphate	TCRE	transcervical resection of endometrium
MRI	magnetic resonance imaging		
MTP	medical termination of pregnancy	TID	thrice daily
		TORCH	toxoplasma, rubella, cytomegalovirus, herpes virus
NSAID	nonsteroidal anti-inflammatory drug	TSH	thyroid stimulating hormone
NST	nonstress test	USG	ultrasonography
OD	once a day	UTI	urinary tract infection
P/A	per abdomen	VDRL	venereal diseases research laboratory (test)
P/R	per rectum		

Contents

CHAPTER 1

Communication with the patient and history-taking

ASHA OUMACHIGUI

The doctors should return to their roots as healers and teachers.

R. Horton

The practice of obstetrics and gynecology requires a number of skills. In addition to knowledge and practical skills, a doctor should develop interpersonal communication skills that help build up a doctor–patient relationship, and trust, which is the essence of clinical medicine. A patient presents with a 'problem' that needs to be analysed, keeping in mind the 'whole patient'; good communication helps the patient to relax and enables the doctor to gain her confidence. For many patients, especially women, consulting a doctor is an ordeal as bad as a viva voce is for students. Once the patient is put at ease, the doctor may 'listen to the patient telling him the diagnosis'.

Objectives

At the end of this chapter, the reader should be able to

- ❑ Define communication.
- ❑ Enumerate the principles of good communication.
- ❑ Appreciate that good communication is essential to the practice of obstetrics and gynecology.
- ❑ Elicit an accurate account of the symptoms.
- ❑ Assess the patient's problem against her family and social background.
- ❑ Interpret the information in the light of the patient's problem.
- ❑ Appreciate that history-taking is an essential step towards management of the patient.

COMMUNICATION

Definition

Communication is derived from the Latin word *communis*, which means common, or general. When we communicate, we try to find something in common between ourselves and the person(s) with whom we are communicating.

Communication is a process. It is dynamic, as it changes depending on what the person with whom one is communicating says. It involves the transfer and sharing of meanings. It is the *people* involved in the communication process who give meaning to words, body language or symbols. It is important to understand that communication is not possible without perception, that is, the process of forming impressions about a person or an event and then making a judgement about it.

When communication is poor, the message received is very different from the message sent (Fig. 1.1). The message sent and the message received are the same if communication is good. There is a need therefore, to understand the principles of good communication.

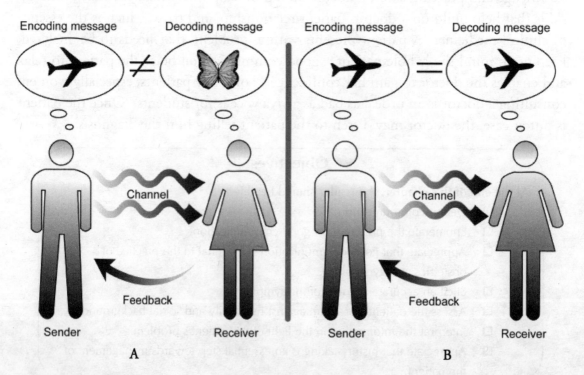

Fig. 1.1 The communication model. A: Poor communication; B: Good communication

Principles of good communication

Patients consult a doctor on their own, but they also believe that doctors are 'formidable'. In the context of rural India, many consider doctors next to god. This is evident in the respectful way they enter a doctor's consultation room. If the doctor is rude, patients are frightened and unable to communicate (Fig. 1.2).

In obstetrics and gynecology, the questions asked are related to genital organs, sexual function and loss of pregnancy, all of which are not only personal, but also likely to disturb a patient emotionally. Therefore, establishing a good rapport with the patient by greeting her and smiling at her, goes a long way in putting her at ease (Fig. 1.2).

It is imperative to demonstrate *empathy*—putting oneself in the patient's position. The doctor's gestures and facial expression should assure the patient that she has the doctor's full attention.

Every doctor must develop the skill of *active listening*. This means not only hearing, but also filtering, interpreting and evaluating the information given by the patient. The doctor must show interest by responding and asking questions in an interested

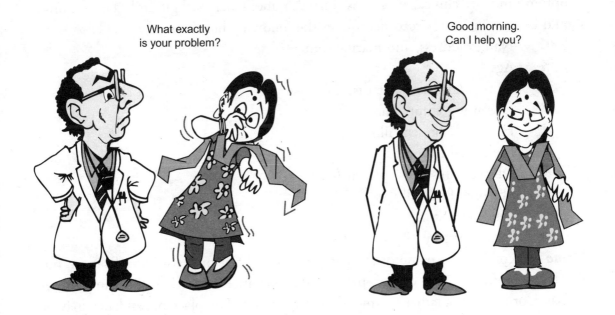

Fig. 1.2 A rude doctor frightens patients away,
while a sympathetic doctor puts the patient at ease.

way. When a patient talks, both the words and gestures the doctor uses are important. She must be allowed to tell the story in her own words and in any sequence as far as possible, since each patient may explain her problems in a different way. Her communication is influenced by age, familial context, sociocultural background, educational status and above all, her personality. Most importantly, the doctor must make the patient feel that he is interested in her welfare, in order to build up a relationship of trust.

Once such a relationship is established, the patient is inclined to provide information about herself readily and to understand the implications of subjecting herself to the different choices of investigative and treatment protocols. Last, but not the least, good communication is likely to minimise litigation and so, in his own interest, a doctor should acquire communication skills and develop a good rapport with the patient.

HISTORY-TAKING

The aim of history-taking is to elicit relevant information not only about the patient's symptoms and her clinical problems, but also about her background. The findings should be conventionally recorded under the following headings:

❖   Name, address, and marital status
❖   Age
❖   Occupation, social status, literacy
❖   Presenting complaints
❖   History of present illness
❖   Menstrual history
❖   Obstetric history—present/past
❖   History of past illness
❖   Personal history
❖   Family history

Name—Recording the name of the patient is useful not only for identification, but also in promoting a good doctor–patient relationship. If married, the name of her husband, or if not, the father's name, should be noted. The place of residence may be urban or rural; it indicates the availability of health care facilities or whether the area is endemic for diseases like malaria. All these environmental factors have a bearing on the patient's problems either directly or indirectly.

Age—Several gynecological disorders are strongly related to age. For example, ovarian cancer and uterovaginal prolapse occur commonly in the postmenopausal period, while fibroids are encountered in the reproductive age group. Pregnancy in girls of 18 years or less and in women of 35 years or more, is more likely to be associated with complications.

Occupation, socioeconomic status and literacy—It is now well recognised that the occupation from which a patient earns her livelihood has an important influence on her health status. Hookworm infestation is more prevalent among labourers who work barefoot, and is an important cause of anemia in India.

Epidemiological studies have shown that diseases like malnutrition, tuberculosis (TB) and rheumatic heart disease occur more frequently in individuals from the lower socioeconomic class.

Literacy has been found to be an important determinant of desirable health seeking behaviour.

Presenting complaints—An attempt should be made to define the presenting complaint and its duration. The presenting complaint is simply the complaint which makes the patient seek a doctor's help. Due to the very personal nature of the problem, a patient may not present with the actual complaint. For example, stigma is attached to childlessness, and talking about one's sexual problems is taboo; therefore the patient, not infrequently, presents with abdominal pain or backache. In such cases, the doctor needs to patiently win her confidence before the person decides to reveal the real problem.

In some cases, the patient may have several other complaints; these too must be recorded chronologically. It is difficult to elicit the duration of the problem among the elderly, the illiterate and the poor. However, on persistent inquiry, they might be able to relate the onset of the problem with special occasions like festivals, or an important event in the family. It may not be out of place to mention that women who have undergone tubectomy relate every complaint to the procedure. It helps to ask *'when were you perfectly alright?'* The patient would then respond with reference to the above points.

History of present illness—Once the doctor is able to guess the nature of the problem, direct questions regarding history of present illness should be asked as follows:
1. Treatment taken earlier for a similar complaint is important. Its effectiveness should be ascertained.

2. Alteration in functions of other systems: Dyspepsia, loss of appetite, vomiting and alteration in bowel movements may be the main complaint in case of ovarian cancer or a very large ovarian tumour.

3. Urinary system: Difficulty in initiation of micturition is associated with uterovaginal prolapse.

4. A note must be made if the patient is on treatment for diabetes mellitus, bronchial asthma, hypertension and epilepsy.

Menstrual history—Every woman should be asked about her *menstruation.* In the majority of women, the duration of the menstrual cycle is 28 days; the menstrual flow lasts for 3–4 days and amounts to 50–80 ml. The presence of clots in menstrual flow indicates excessive bleeding. Regular cycles are suggestive of ovulation. The doctor must also enquire about pain associated with menstruation; colicky pain during menstruation suggests submucous fibroid. The onset of pain with menstruation later in life is suggestive of a fibroid uterus or endometriosis.

Noting the date of the first day of the last menstrual period (LMP) is necessary in order to plan certain gynecological procedures and also to calculate the expected date of delivery (EDD).

Obstetric history—Accurate recording of *obstetric history,* both present and past is invaluable for decision-making in obstetrics. A doctor is generally called upon to answer three questions: (i) What is the period of gestation? (ii) At what period of gestation should the pregnancy be terminated? (iii) How should the pregnancy be terminated?

At the outset, the doctor must enquire about parity, abortions, live children and the order of pregnancy. Frequently, the presenting complaint is not amenorrhea, especially in the later half of gestation, by which time most women realise that they are pregnant. The complaint is often a manifestation of pregnancy complications such as swelling of feet in pre-eclampsia, or associated diseases like anemia or heart disease. Occasionally, they may present with abdominal pain attributable to onset of labour, gynecologic or surgical disorders.

When a pregnant mother consults a doctor, the following information must be sought.

First trimester
i) Date and method of confirmation of pregnancy. This is very useful in assessing the period of gestation.

ii) Complaints such as excessive vomiting, bleeding per vaginum, history suggestive of urinary tract infection, fever associated with rash.

iii) History of taking drugs, exposure to radiation with reference to fetal congenital anomalies.

Second trimester

i) Quickening is the first perception of fetal movements by the mother. It is experienced by primigravida around 20 weeks of gestation and by multigravida around 18 weeks of gestation. Most mothers are unable to give the exact date of quickening and hence it may not be reliable in calculating the period of gestation.

ii) History of swelling of lower limbs especially late in the second trimester suggests the possibility of pre-eclampsia. Headache, blurred vision and oliguria point to the presence of imminent eclampsia and not just pre-eclampsia.

iii) Bleeding per vaginum could be due to low lying placenta or separation of a normally situated placenta.

Third trimester

i) In this trimester, it is mandatory to ask for the features of pre-eclampsia mentioned above.

ii) Enquire about bleeding.

iii) Enquiry must be made about antenatal care received so far.

A record of the number of antenatal visits should be made. In India, minimum antenatal care is qualified by four visits, with one visit each in the first and second trimester, and two visits in the last trimester. The reason for advocating two visits in the last trimester is to detect conditions like pregnancy induced hypertension (PIH) abnormal presentations and cephalopelvic disproportion. One must gather information regarding weight gain, blood pressure, immunisation against tetanus, iron folic acid prophylaxis and drugs taken for any illness. It is worthwhile to ascertain whether an ultrasonography was performed at 16–18 weeks for morphological study of the fetus. The results of investigations, such as blood group and Rh typing, hemoglobin, urinalysis, VDRL and any other relevant tests should be noted.

Past obstetric history should be recorded. While eliciting history, follow an established order—date of delivery, duration of pregnancy, health during pregnancy, place of delivery, personnel who conducted the delivery, type of delivery (whether spontaneous vaginal, operative vaginal or cesarean section). If operative, one must try and ascertain the indication for operative intervention. Enquiry must be made regarding the nature of anesthesia administered, intra- and postoperative complications, history of blood transfusion and duration of hospital stay.

Detailed information should be obtained about the baby—whether born alive, cried at birth, weight and sex of the baby, whether congenital anomalies were present and corrected. If the baby was stillborn, attempt should be made to ascertain the cause. If the fetal heart sound disappeared during labour, it could be due to intrapartum asphyxia; antepartum hemorrhage and severe pre-eclampsia could lead to fetal death before onset of labour. Occasionally, a cord accident may be responsible for stillbirth.

Whenever there is a history of abortion, one should find out the period of gestation and whether it was spontaneous; if it occurred spontaneously, preceded by glairy mucus discharge and not much pain, the cause of abortion could be incompetent os. Early abortions may be attributed to cytogenetic abnormalities. If the abortion was induced, one should check the methods used and any complications that ensued.

History of previous illness—The patient must be asked about all the diseases she had prior to the present illness or pregnancy. Particular attention must be paid to diseases like TB, reproductive tract infection (RTI), sexually transmitted diseases (STD), and rheumatic fever. These could be causally related to the present illness; the presence of RTI, STD, or TB in the past may be responsible for infertility. Previous history of jaundice may point to hepatic dysfunction and could be a contraindication to the use of oral contraceptives. Past history of trauma, surgery, type of anesthesia and blood transfusion may be associated with sequelae or may warn the doctor to anticipate difficulties while administering anesthesia or performing surgery.

Personal history—One must elicit information regarding addiction to tobacco (smoking/chewing), alcohol and hard drugs. These addictions are associated with intrauterine growth restriction (IUGR) and other adverse perinatal outcomes.

One should next ask about the diet with reference to intake of calories, protein, calcium and other essential nutrients.

It is not uncommon to encounter individuals who are allergic to certain drugs. A note must be made of these drugs. The allergic reaction can sometimes be life-threatening. Therefore, if a patient is allergic to a particular drug, it should be noted prominently on the case sheet.

Family history—Some diseases like essential hypertension, diabetes mellitus, bleeding disorders, and breast cancer are hereditary. Tuberculosis and STD may be transmitted through proximity. If there has been a death in the family, one must ascertain the cause of death.

In an obstetric case, in addition to the disorders mentioned above, one must enquire about pre-eclampsia, multiple pregnancy and congenital anomalies, especially in the mother or sisters.

Developing a good rapport with the patient helps a doctor gather useful information regarding her problems. These details are useful not only for arriving at a diagnosis, but also for choosing the right option for management of the problem for which the patient has consulted the doctor.

Key points

1. Interpersonal communication skills are essential to build up a good doctor–patient relationship.
2. Communication is a dynamic process which involves transfer and sharing of meanings.
3. The key to good communication is active listening.
4. History-taking is necessary to elicit information about the patient's problems and her background.
5. The information gathered must be recorded systematically and interpreted in the light of the patient's problem.
6. A carefully recorded history is useful not only for arriving at a clinical diagnosis, but also for ensuring the patient's compliance with the treatment.

CHAPTER 2

General physical examination

S. HABEEBULLAH

General physical examination forms an important part of the examination of a patient. It may not only give clues about the underlying disease process, but also help in assessing the severity of the problem with which the patient presents. The findings of general examination could also influence the selection of treatment options.

Objectives

At the end of this chapter, the reader should be able to

- ❑ Appreciate the importance of general physical examination in an obstetric and gynecologic patient.
- ❑ Elicit various signs.
- ❑ Correlate the signs with the possible underlying clinical condition.

COMPONENTS OF THE EXAMINATION

The *general condition* should be assessed. It is important to note whether the patient is conscious, drowsy or comatose. Orientation to time and place, and response to commands should also be evaluated. This is relevant to patients with eclampsia, septicemia, cortical vein thrombosis, shock, intracranial hemorrhage and postpartum psychosis.

The height and weight parameters, to some extent, reflect the nutritional status of the patient. Upto 40 per cent of short statured women (≤ 140 cm) may have a generally contracted pelvis with an increased risk of cephalopelvic disproportion. Very tall women are likely to have an anthropoid type of pelvis. Short stature is also a prominent feature of pituitary disorders and Turner syndrome, which may present as primary amenorrhea. Based on height and weight, one can calculate body mass index (BMI = weight in kg ÷ height in m²). BMI of more than 26 indicates obesity which may be associated with diabetes mellitus or hypothyroidism. These patients are prone to problems during anesthesia, operative procedures and postoperative complications. Low BMI (less than 19) indicates poor nutritional status, which may be associated with anemia, intrauterine growth restriction (IUGR) and malignancies. Serial recording of weight in a pregnant patient helps in early identification of pregnancy induced hypertension (PIH) and anticipation of IUGR.

The weight of the patient is also taken into account while administering drugs like chemotherapeutic agents.

❖ Facial *appearance* may reflect the underlying disease, like systemic lupus erythematosus (SLE), Cushing's disease or hyperthyroidism.

❖ Assessment of *hydration* is important in patients who have vomiting as in hyperemesis gravidarum, gastroenteritis, acute pain in abdomen, following chemotherapy and those who are on exclusive intravenous (IV) therapy.

❖ *Pallor* is evident over facial skin, palpebral conjunctiva, nail bed and vaginal mucosa. Anemia can be nutritional, or due to acute or chronic bleeding. It has important bearing on pregnancy. Severe anemia is an indication for hospitalisation and blood transfusion. Conditions like abortion, ectopic pregnancy, antepartum hemorrhage (APH) and postpartum hemorrhage (PPH), menorrhagia, hemorrhoids and genital tract malignancy predispose a woman to anemia.

❖ In obstetrics, *icterus* may be seen in severe pre-eclampsia, eclampsia, hyperemesis gravidarum and associated hepatitis. It can also be drug-induced (anti-TB drugs), or due to secondaries in liver caused by malignancies.

❖ *Cyanosis* is generally seen in cardiac disease complicating pregnancy, in eclampsia due to continuous convulsions or aspiration, and in severe respiratory diseases.

❖ Pregnancy *per se* is associated with some degree of tachycardia. A rise in *pulse* rate indicates the presence of infection, fever or loss of fluid or blood. An irregular pulse reflects cardiac complications.

❖ *Blood pressure* (BP) should be recorded routinely in all pregnant women at every visit, in order to detect PIH at the earliest. The criteria to diagnose PIH are either a rise of 15 mm Hg in diastolic BP and 30 mm Hg in systolic BP or recording an absolute value of 140/90 or above on two occasions six hours apart.

A fall in BP is noted in case of shock due to dehydration, hemorrhage and septicemia; it requires immediate institution of resuscitative measures.

❖ Physiological *edema* is noted in about 40 per cent of pregnant women. Edema which does not subside after a night's rest is pathological. Besides facial puffiness, edema of hands and abdomen should be considered pathological. It may be present in PIH, cardiac disease with failure, severe anemia with hypoproteinemia or with congestive cardiac failure, in renal failure and cirrhosis of the liver.

Unilateral edema of lower limb may be seen in filariasis, venous thrombosis, lymph node involvement in malignant ovarian tumour or cancer vulva, and due to lymphedema following radical surgery with lymphadenectomy and radiotherapy. Supraclavicular, axillary, paraaortic, iliac and groin nodes may be enlarged in different genital tract and breast malignancies. Matted lymph node enlargement may also be seen in TB.

❖ *Thyromegaly* should be looked for especially in adolescent girls with menorrhagia, infertility and recurrent abortions.

❖ *Hirsutism* is present in polycystic ovarian syndrome (PCOS). Severe degree of hirsutism is associated with androgen-producing tumours of the ovary.

❖ *Breasts* must be examined routinely in all women so as to detect a lump, even when they are asymptomatic.

  a. In early pregnancy, breasts show fullness, vascular prominence and Montgomery tubercles with pigmentation of primary areola and appearance of secondary areola. Nipples should be inspected for any retraction, cracks or ulcers. These should be treated antenatally for successful breast feeding.

  b. In women presenting with amenorrhea and infertility, the breasts should be examined to note the development – Tanner staging. One should look for galactorrhea, which may be seen in disorders like hyperprolactinemia and hypothyroidism.

❖ *Temperature*—Fever is an important sign of underlying infections like urinary tract infection (UTI), chorio-amnionitis, puerperal sepsis, septic abortion and eclampsia (following convulsion) and endocarditis. Temperature can be low in cases of septic shock.

It is important to remember that a proper general examination is essential in order to develop a holistic approach to the management of women presenting with problems related to the reproductive tract.

Key points

1. General examination is an essential component of physical examination.
2. The findings are useful in assessing the severity of the underlying disease.
3. The information obtained could influence the choice of treatment.

CHAPTER 3

Gynecologic and obstetric examination

GITA RAJAGOPALAN
ASHA OUMACHIGUI

Use technology to confirm your diagnosis, rather than to rule it out.

A thorough history and general physical examination must always precede gynecologic and obstetric examination. The information thus obtained is useful not only in assessing the general condition of the patient, but may also give a clue to the problem with which the patient has presented. Also, the physical examination is performed against this background. Examination of the breasts, abdomen and pelvis are essential parts of a gynecologic examination. In the majority of cases, a diagnosis can be made from the information obtained from history and physical examination. Relevant investigations can then be selected to (i) assess the general health status of the patient, (ii) confirm the clinical diagnosis, (iii) assess severity of the disease, and (iv) detect complications.

Objectives

At the end of this chapter, the reader should be able to

- ❏ Appreciate the need to perform a complete physical examination.
- ❏ Ensure that essential prerequisites are fulfilled before an abdominal or pelvic examination is performed.
- ❏ Describe the procedure for examination of the abdomen.
- ❏ Describe the steps in pelvic examination.
- ❏ Describe the steps in obstetric examination and a normal fetopelvic relation.
- ❏ Recollect the purpose of pelvic examination in obstetrics.

PREREQUISITES

Examination of a gynecologic case is essentially concerned with the examination of genitalia. Therefore, absolute privacy must be ensured before beginning the examination. There should be good light for inspection of the abdomen, external genitalia and more importantly, for satisfactory viewing of the vagina and the cervix. A full bladder may vitiate the estimation of the uterine size; the patient is therefore requested to void urine before she lies on the couch. The nature of the examination must be explained to her. *The presence of a female attendant is mandatory when a male doctor examines the patient.*

Breast

During pregnancy, there is an increase in size and vascularity of the breast. Raised nodules appear in the areolar region, which are in essence, sebaceous glands and are called Montgomery's tubercles. Later on, there is darkening of the areola and pigmentation around the areola, which is called the secondary areola.

The nipples should be examined for retraction, and if found, measures should be taken for correction. If left uncorrected, it can lead to difficulty in feeding and subsequently, to breast engorgement. For further details of breast examination see Chapter 34.

Abdomen

The patient should be in the *dorsal position* with lower limbs extended. The whole abdomen must be exposed, taking care to cover the patient above the xiphisternum and below the upper half of thighs.

A visual inspection must be done. A note must be made of the presence of striae gravidarum, linea nigra or scars of previous surgery. The patient should then be asked to cough in order to detect incisional hernia if a scar is present, one must look for hernia in the umbilical and inguinal regions. If there are any skin lesions, infective or vascular, they must be recorded.

The umbilicus is normally situated between the tip of the xiphoid process and the upper margin of symphysis pubis. It can be displaced by ascites or intraabdominal swelling.

The contour of the abdomen is generally retracted in thin individuals. Symmetrical distension could be due to fat, fluid, flatus, feces or fetus. Distension or tumour of an organ will lead to a localised abdominal distension. In case of a large ovarian cyst, multifetal pregnancy, or pregnancy with polyhydramnios, the abdomen is likely to be extremely distended, with the umbilicus flattened or everted and the skin stretched and shiny.

Palpation—The patient is requested to flex the lower limbs at the knees and hips, to ensure relaxation of abdominal muscles and is asked to breathe quietly. At this stage, the doctor must reassure the patient that the examination will be done as gently as possible. If the patient has pain at a particular site, it should be palpated last.

Palpation is the most important part of the abdominal examination. It must be performed gently, but with firm pressure, with fingers almost straight with slight flexion at the metacarpophalangeal joints. All the quadrants of the abdomen should be palpated. In the upper quadrant, one must look for enlargement of the liver, spleen and gall bladder; metastatic deposits in the omentum can sometimes be felt as a fairly large lump.

When there is a mass in the lower abdomen, it is most likely to arise from the uterus or the ovary, and less commonly, from the appendix, cecum or the fallopian tube. For details of examination of a lower abdominal mass see Chapter 32.

Sometimes an ovarian cyst may grow large enough to occupy the whole abdomen and may be confused with ascites. These two conditions can be differentiated by percussion:

Ovarian cyst—The note is dull around the umbilicus and resonant in the flanks.

Ascites—The note is resonant in the centre and dull in the flanks when the patient is supine. If she is made to lie on her side, the upper flank is resonant. This 'shifting dullness' is characteristic of free fluid in the peritoneal cavity, whatever be the underlying pathology.

PELVIC EXAMINATION

The procedure should be explained to the patient. She is asked to flex the knee and hip joints completely. Before commencing the examination, the doctor must wear gloves on both hands. The components of this examination are described below.

Inspection of external genitalia—Inspection of the mons pubis, labia majora, labia minora, perineal body and the anal region is performed to check the contour, skin lesions, distribution of the hair or any swelling. If there is any swelling, it should be palpated. The labia are separated to inspect the introitus and the clitoris. The patient is asked to strain to see if there is any cystocele or rectocele. The external urinary meatus should also be inspected.

Speculum examination for visualisation of the cervix and the vagina is an essential part of gynecologic examination. Several vaginal specula are available. However, the most commonly used ones are the bivalved Cusco's or the single or double ended Sims' speculum; an anterior vaginal retractor must be used along with the Sims' speculum, especially if the anterior vaginal wall is lax and the cervix cannot be viewed.

The patient may either continue to be in the dorsal position or may be shifted to left lateral position. The procedure is explained to the patient. Then, the moistened speculum is held in the right hand, and using the index finger and the thumb of the left hand, the labia are separated, the speculum is inserted into the vagina with the blade in an oblique direction and pressed against the perineum, and then rotated gently to the transverse plane on the posterior vaginal wall (Fig. 3.1). The position of the speculum is adjusted till the cervix and the vagina can be viewed.

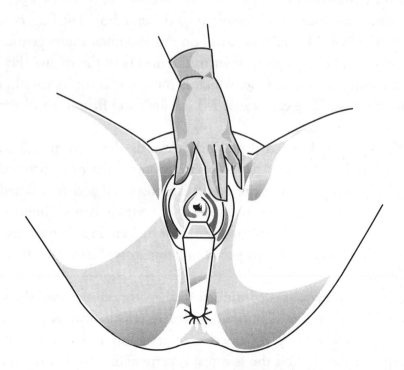

Fig. 3.1 Speculum examination

The purpose of this examination is to inspect the vagina and the cervix for the following:

❖ Presence of blood
❖ Presence of discharge; its colour and character are noted. The discharge should be collected and examined microscopically.
❖ The ectocervix is inspected for the presence of bluish discolouration associated with pregnancy (Chadwick sign) and a similar change in the vagina (Jacquemier sign).

A note should be made about the presence of lesions on the cervix and the vagina; they could be infective (ulcers), neoplastic (cancer of the cervix) or traumatic (lacerations). **A Pap smear should be taken** before proceeding to the bimanual examination.

Bimanual pelvic examination—One hand should be placed on the lower abdomen and the lubricated fingers (middle and index) of the other hand are inserted in the vagina. The examining fingers are kept away from the clitoris and urethral meatus in order to **avoid discomfort** to the patient; pressure should be exerted on the perineal body until the perineal muscles are relaxed (Figs 3.2 and 3.3). The fingers are advanced along the posterior vaginal wall. The hand on the abdomen exerts gentle, downward pressure bringing the pelvic organs closer to the fingers in the vagina (Fig. 3.4). The cervix is then identified by a dimple, which is the external os; its length, consistency and direction are noted. The cervix is 2.5–3 cm long and firm in consistency. During pregnancy, the cervix is soft.

In general, the os is directed posteriorly towards the sacrum and the uterus is anteverted and anteflexed (Fig. 3.5). In many women, the os is directed anteriorly, towards the symphysis pubis and the uterus is retroverted and retroflexed (Fig. 3.6). It must be remembered that a retroversion of the uterus is not abnormal unless its mobility is restricted. The cervix is normally mobile by 1 cm in all directions. Tenderness on movement of cervix is present in pelvic inflammatory disease (PID) and disturbed ectopic pregnancy.

The bimanual examination is continued further to note the size, shape, regularity and consistency of the uterus. The nonpregnant uterus is firm. A pregnant uterus is uniformly enlarged and soft. At 8–10 weeks of gestation, the products of conception are lodged near the fundus and the isthmus is extremely soft with the result that the fingers in the vagina appear to meet the fingers on the abdomen. This is known as

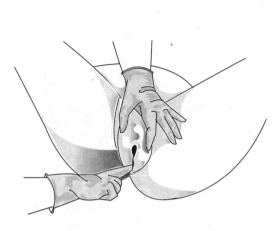

Fig. 3.2 Steps in bimanual examination:
Introduction of index finger into vagina

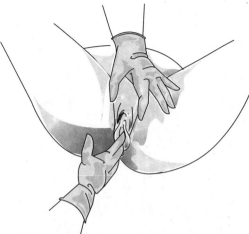

Fig. 3.3 Steps in bimanual examination:
Introduction of index and middle fingers
into vagina

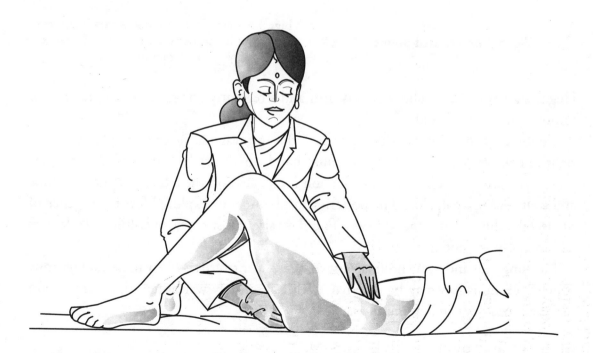

Fig. 3.4 Steps in bimanual examination: The other hand is placed over the lower abdomen

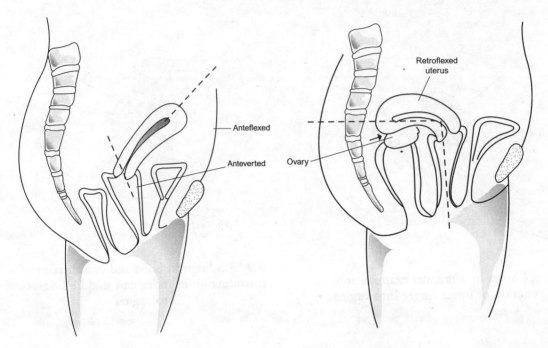

Fig. 3.5 Anterverted uterus

Fig. 3.6 Retroflexed uterus: Arrow denotes ovary impinged between retroflexed uterus and rectum

Hegar sign (Fig. 3.7). The uterus is firm and irregularly enlarged in the presence of tumour (such as a fibroid).

Continuing the bimanual examination, the intravaginal fingers are placed in the right lateral fornix, while the abdominal hand on the right lower quadrant exerts downward pressure. Then the examination is repeated on the left side. A normal tube and ovary are not palpable. The posterior fornix must be explored for the presence of a mass or nodules. If an adnexal mass is found, its size, consistency, pulsaltility, tenderness and mobility are noted.

In young girls and some nulliparous women, the introitus is likely to be very narrow. A pelvic examination may be deferred, and if absolutely warranted, the examination may be carried out under anesthesia.

Rectal examination
The perianal and anal region should be inspected for any lesions due to scratching, presence of piles, fissures and fistulae.

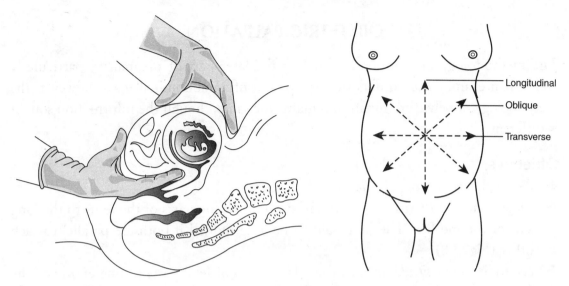

Fig. 3.7 Hegar sign   **Fig. 3.8 Abdominal examination: lie of the fetus**

The anal canal and rectum are palpated with a gloved, well-lubricated index finger. A tight external sphincter and tenderness are characteristic of anal fissure or painful hemorrhoids. On rectal examination, one can evaluate more easily a mass or nodules in the pouch of Douglas. Infiltration of the parametria is appreciated better on rectal examination.

The cervix, uterus and adnexal mass can be evaluated through the anterior rectal wall in women in whom vaginal examination cannot be performed.

OBSTETRIC EXAMINATION

The clinical features of early pregnancy by pelvic examination have already been described. Performing a pelvic examination in early pregnancy has the following advantages:

* The uterine enlargement corresponds fairly accurately with the period of gestation. This information is useful if there is a doubt about the dates.
* Associated *lesions* on the cervix and vagina can be viewed.
* The presence of *adnexal* tumours or fibroids can be appreciated.
* *Ectopic pregnancy* can be excluded.
* Helps to recognise the *type of abortions*.
* An *incompetent os* can be detected.

OBSTETRIC PALPATION

The methodology of examination during the later part of pregnancy, particularly abdominal examination, differs from palpation of an abdominal mass; however, the methodology of pelvic examination remains the same, though the information sought is different.

Objectives

❖ Assess the *period of gestation.*
❖ Detect the *lie of fetus,* that is, the relation of the long axis of the fetus to the long axis of the mother. The lie is said to be longitudinal if both are parallel to each other (Fig. 3.8).
❖ Ascertain the *attitude,* that is, the relationship of fetal parts to one another. The fetus is normally in a state of universal flexion. In certain cases, there may be deflexion or extension of the fetal head (Fig. 3.9).
❖ Detect the *presentation,* that is, the fetal part occupying the lower pole of the uterus.

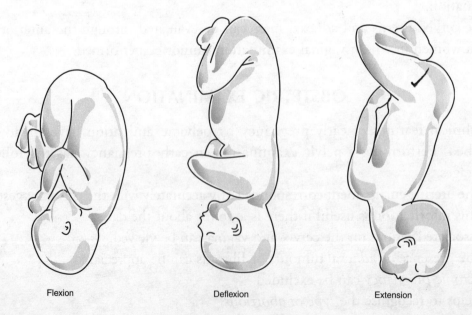

Flexion   Deflexion   Extension

Fig. 3.9 Attitude of fetal head

❖ *Position* refers to the relationship of a fixed point on the presenting part, known as the denominator, to fixed points on the maternal pelvis. For example, the occiput is the denominator in a vertex presentation. The position can be determined by the location of the fetal spine and the anterior shoulder from the midline; on vaginal examination, the position can be confirmed by the location of the posterior fontanelle to fixed points on the pelvis like the symphysis pubis, ileopectineal eminence, sacroiliac joint and the sacral promontory (Fig. 3.10).

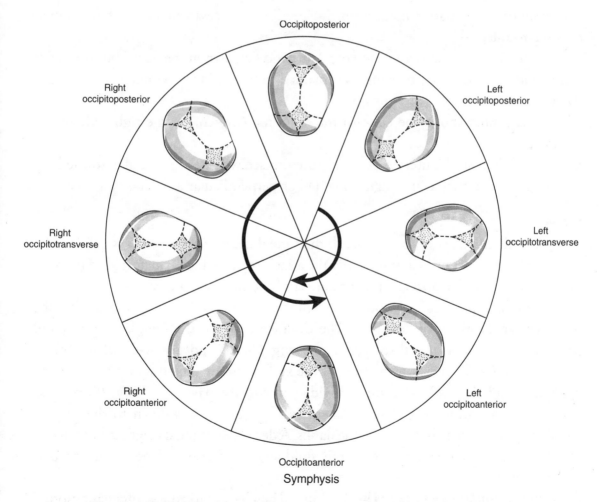

Fig. 3.10 Various positions of vertex at onset of labour. Arrows indicate degree of rotation needed to reach occipitoanterior position

❖ Assess the *level of the fetal presenting part in relation to the pelvic brim*—The head is engaged if the biparietal diameter has crossed the pelvic brim.

❖ Evaluate *fetal size.*

❖ Identify uterine contractions.

❖ Obstetric examination must be performed systematically towards gathering the above information, which is required to make two important decisions in obstetrics, particularly in high-risk cases, regarding *termination* of pregnancy.

   a.   *When* should a pregnancy be terminated?

   b.   What should be the *mode* of termination?

Any significant observation made during inspection like a cesarean scar on the abdomen must be recollected.

The pregnant mother is asked to void urine and lie down in the dorsal position with legs partially flexed. The procedure is explained to her and the abdomen is exposed as described earlier.

❖ The examiner should be close to the examining couch, on the right side of the patient.

❖ The contour of the uterine ovoid is noted to see whether it is parallel to the long axis of the mother as in longitudinal lie, or perpendicular as in transverse lie.

Steps

Using the ulnar border of the left hand, the fundal height of the uterus is palpated by passing the hand from below upwards till a lack of resistance is detected. The right hand of the examiner corrects dextrorotation of the uterus if present.

The uterus is palpable just above the symphysis pubis at 12 weeks and reaches the umbilicus at 24 weeks of gestation. The distance between the symphysis pubis and umbilicus is divided into three parts, marking 16, 20 and 24 weeks of gestation. At 36 weeks, the fundus is at the level of the xiphisternum. The distance between the umbilicus and the xiphisternum is divided into three parts, marking 28, 32 and 36 weeks of gestation (Fig. 3.11). At term, the fundus comes down to the level of costal margin and there is fullness of the flanks. A decrease in fundal height is attributable to a decrease in the quantity of amniotic fluid and the descent of the presenting part into the pelvis.

Symphysio fundal height (SFH)—The fundal height is marked, the pregnant mother then extends the lower limbs to avoid errors due to tilting of pelvis. The distance between symphysis pubis and the fundal height is measured in centimeters. Ideally, the SFH is measured throughout pregnancy and the values are plotted on a gravidogram to monitor fetal growth. If the measurements are below the 50th percentile, IUGR must be suspected and the patient should be referred for further fetal evaluation. Thus, the gravidogram is a good screening method for IUGR (Fig. 3.12). A single measurement in centimeters corresponds to the gestational age in weeks between 18 and 30 weeks.

Fundal grip—The examiner faces the patient and places both hands on the uterine fundus. In a cephalic presentation, the breech is felt at the fundus. It is felt as a broad based, irregular and nonballotable mass (Fig. 3.13a).

Lateral umbilical grip—The examiner's hands are placed on the flanks, on either side of the umbilicus and one hand steadies the fetus while the other hand palpates. In a

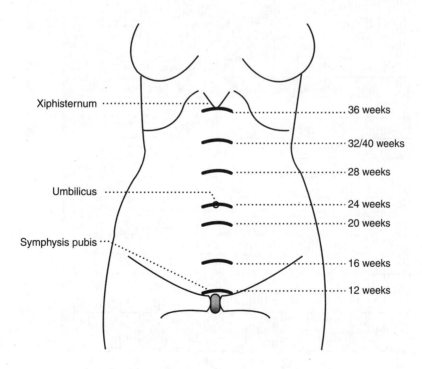

Fig. 3.11 Fundal height and gestational age

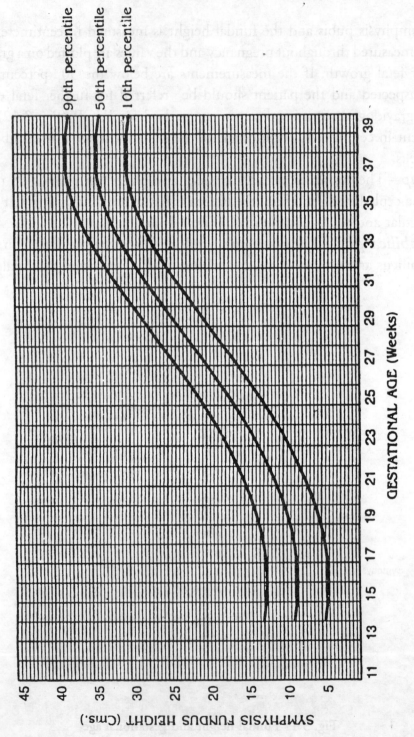

Fig. 3.12 Gravidogram: maternal symphysis-fundus growth chart

longitudinal lie, the smooth curve of the back is felt on one side while irregular nodular limb buds are felt on the opposite side (Fig. 3.13b).

First pelvic grip (Pawlik's grip)—The thumb and four fingers are placed over the lower pole of the uterus with the ulnar border of the examiner's hand being placed over the symphysis pubis. The presenting part is grasped and its side-to-side mobility is assessed. In a cephalic presentation, the head is felt as a hard, globular and ballotable mass (Fig. 3.13c). First pelvic grip also helps to recognise whether the head is engaged; when the head is engaged, either the sinciput alone, or no part of the head, is palpable. This information is useful in monitoring the descent of the head during labour (Fig. 3.14).

Second pelvic grip—The examiner stands facing the feet of the patient. Either hand is placed on the lower abdomen parallel to the inguinal ligament, the cephalic pole is palpated and the occiput and sinciput are felt (Fig. 3.13d). The occiput is a broad and smooth prominence felt on the same side as the back of the fetus, as compared to the sinciput, which is smaller and sharper. The attitude of the fetal head can be appreciated. If the head is well flexed, the occiput is felt at a lower level than the sinciput. If the head is deflexed, both the cephalic eminences are at the same level and if the fetal head is extended, the occiput is felt at a higher level than the sinciput.

Auscultation of fetal heart sound—This should be done at the junction of the lateral third and medial two-thirds of a line joining the umbilicus to the anterior superior iliac spine (spino-umbilical line), in a vertex anterior position, on the side of the back of the fetus, as this is where the fetal heart beat is heard best. In occipitoposterior position, the fetal heart sounds are heard laterally in the flanks or towards the midline. In a breech presentation, the heart sounds are heard higher up at the level of the umbilicus.

BIMANUAL EXAMINATION IN LATE PREGNANCY

The purpose of performing a bimanual examination is to
* Confirm the diagnosis of labour
* Assess cephalopelvic disproportion
* Monitor labour

On bimanual examination, the following criteria confirm the diagnosis of labour.
* Presence of 'show', that is, blood stained mucus discharge.

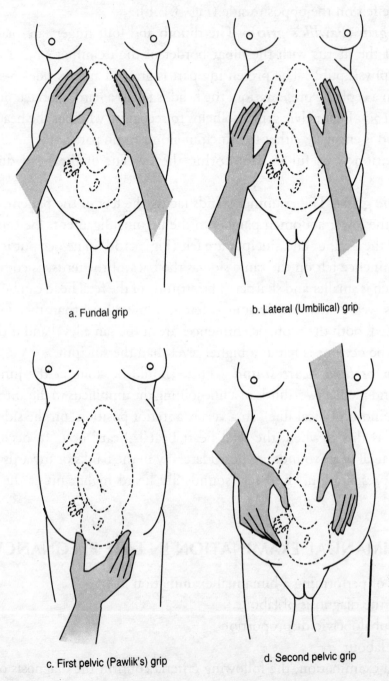

a. Fundal grip

b. Lateral (Umbilical) grip

c. First pelvic (Pawlik's) grip

d. Second pelvic grip

Fig. 3.13 Steps in obsteric palpation

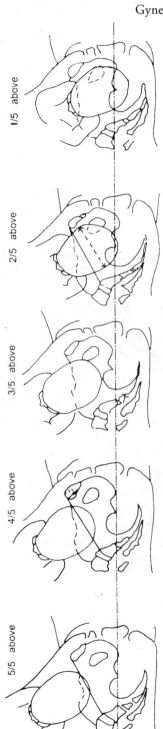

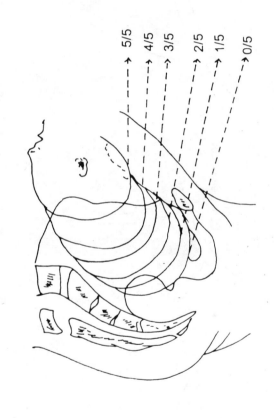

Fig. 3.14 Descent of fetal head as assessed on obstetric palpation

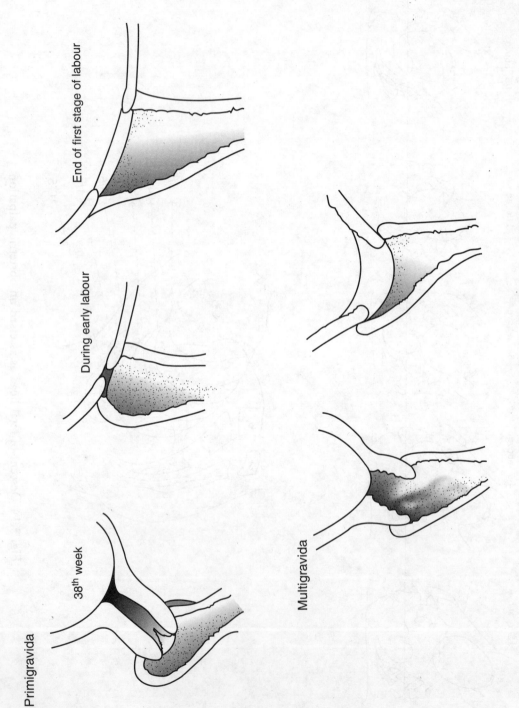

Fig. 3.15 In primigravida, effacement occurs before cervical dilatation.
In multigravida, effacement and cervical dilatation occur simultaneously.

❖ Effacement of cervix and dilatation of cervix of 2–3 cm (Fig. 3.15).

❖ Presence of bag of membranes

In order to evaluate pelvic capacity, one must advance the fingers and try to reach the sacral promontory. If it is reached, the diagonal conjugate can be measured and the anteroposterior diameter of the pelvic inlet is obtained by subtracting 1.5–2 cm (Fig. 3.16). Next, the fingers sweep down the sacrum, to assess the curvature from above downwards and from side to side. Then the convergence of pelvic side walls is noted. This is exaggerated in android and anthropoid type of pelvis as compared to a gynecoid type of pelvis. In fact, a gynecoid pelvis can be described as a short segment of a long cone and the android pelvis as the long segment of a short cone (Fig. 3.17).

Exaggerated convergence of side walls, prominent ischial spines and decreased distance between them (bispinous diameter), and width of sacrospinous ligament less than 3.5 cm, point to a mid-pelvic contraction (Fig. 3.18).

At this stage, the station of the presenting part in relation to ischial spines (zero station) is noted (Fig. 3.19). If the level is high, an attempt should be made to

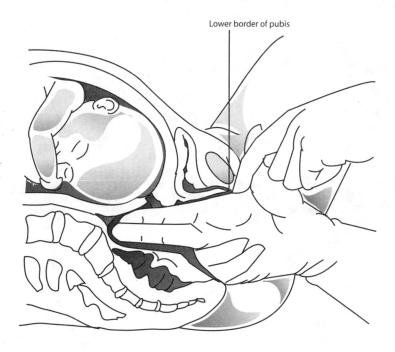

Lower border of pubis

Fig. 3.16 Pelvic assessment: measuring the diagonal conjugate

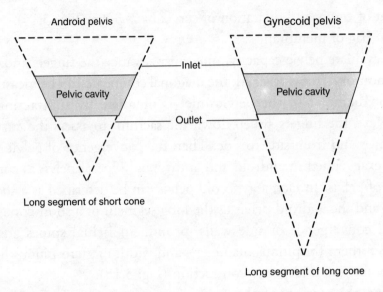

Fig. 3.17 Diagrammatic representation of convergence of side walls and depth of pelvic cavity

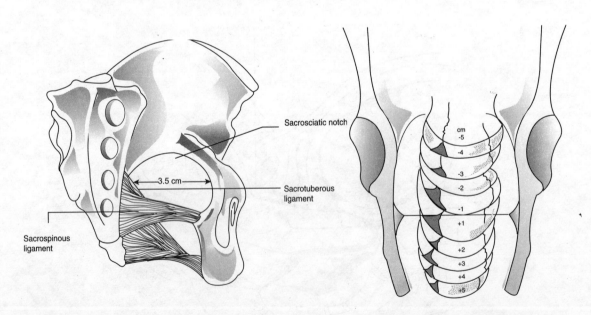

Fig. 3.18 Sacrosciatic notch

Fig. 3.19 Station of the head with reference to ischial spine

push the head per abdomen to see if the presenting part reaches the ischial spines. If it does, the pelvis is said to be adequate.

The examining fingers assess the subpubic arch which is normally rounded. The intertuberous distance is adequate if a clenched hand can be placed between the ischial tuberosities.

The characteristics of an ideal obstetric pelvis (gynecoid) are:

Inlet (Fig. 3.20)

✤ The brim is round or oval transversely.

✤ The anteroposterior diameter is 11 cm.

Cavity

✤ The cavity is shallow.

✤ The sacrum is smoothly curved.

✤ The bispinous diameter is 10 cm.

Outlet (Fig. 3.21)

✤ The subpubic angle is rounded.

✤ The intertuberous diameter is 11 cm.

Bimanual vaginal examination is useful in monitoring labour as it helps to assess progressive dilatation of the cervix and the descent of the presenting part (see Chapter 17).

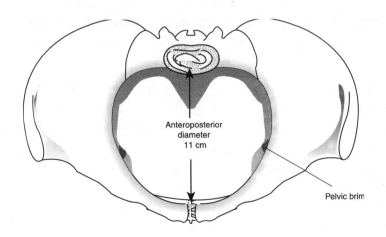

Anteroposterior
diameter
11 cm

Pelvic brim

Fig. 3.20 Gynecoid pelvis

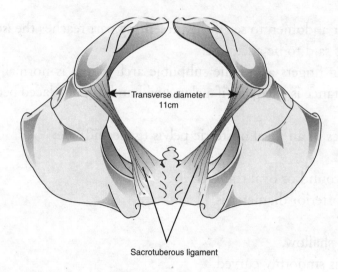

Transverse diameter
11cm

Sacrotuberous ligament

Fig. 3.21 Pelvic outlet

The time-honoured methods of history-taking and physical examination, if properly performed, will make the care of the patient more rational as well as cost effective. Investigations may be performed when required, to help in the diagnosis or management since they are an aid to clinical diagnosis.

Investigations must be selected, performed and interpreted in the light of clinical findings/diagnosis for maximum benefit to the patient. Some investigation procedures are invasive, potentially dangerous and most significantly, expensive.

Key points

1. General physical examination must precede gynecologic and obstetric examination.
2. Good light is essential for proper visualisation of the cervix and the vagina.
3. The nature of the examination should be explained to the patient.
4. The presence of a female attendant is **mandatory** whenever a male doctor examines the patient.
5. Every effort should be made to avoid discomfort to the patient.
6. A clinical diagnosis can be made in most cases using the information obtained from history and physical examination.
7. Investigations must be selected based on the clinical findings.

CHAPTER 4

Care during pregnancy

ASHA OUMACHIGUI

The care of pregnant women started as a social service in Paris in the 18th century. Antenatal care (ANC) as practised currently emerged in the 1960s. Advances in medical sciences in general and technology in particular have contributed effectively to care of the pregnant mother and her child.

The ANC programme is a systematic health care programme for a pregnant mother that involves a coordinated approach to medical, social and psychological management. It should ideally begin before conception and continue till delivery takes place. The overall goals of ANC are to:

1. Evaluate the health of the mother and her fetus.
2. Monitor the progress of pregnancy.
3. Plan further obstetrical care, and mode and timing of delivery.

Objectives

At the end of this chapter, the reader should be able to

- ❑ Define antenatal care (ANC).
- ❑ Enumerate the components of ANC.
- ❑ Assess the duration of gestation.
- ❑ Monitor the health of the mother and her child.
- ❑ Impart comprehensive care according to the national guidelines.
- ❑ Manage minor ailments.
- ❑ Appreciate any deviation from normal.
- ❑ Refer the pregnant mother appropriately for further care or delivery.

CLINICAL SCENARIO

A 25-year-old woman presents with complaint of amenorrhea of 2 months' duration.

HISTORY

 What questions should be asked to acquire more information regarding the symptoms with which the woman has presented?

Whenever a woman in the reproductive age presents with missed periods, one must consider that she is pregnant, until proved otherwise. General information must be gathered (see Chapter 1). However, it may be pertinent to reiterate some relevant issues/elements.

Status—One must enquire about the occupation of the woman. This information could reflect her socioeconomic status, and her health status. Women doing hard manual labour are often undernourished, get no rest, and therefore tend to give birth to low birthweight babies (LBW). It has been documented that those working in situations where pesticides are used suffer from recurrent pregnancy loss.

Violence—Try to assess if the woman is exposed to domestic violence, since this factor influences the pregnancy outcome adversely.

Age—The woman in question is 25 years of age, which is obstetrically favourable. Women below 18 years are at risk of malnutrition, pregnancy induced hypertension, contracted pelvis and psychological and social stress. Those above 35 years of age are likely to be suffering from medical disorders like hypertension and diabetes mellitus; they may have undergone treatment for gynecological and other conditions like cardiac disease.

Menstruation—It is necessary to find out **the first day** of the last menstrual cycle (this is the last menstrual period—LMP) and the length of the menstrual cycle. If the length of the cycle is 28 days, the expected date of delivery (EDD) is calculated by adding 7 days to the LMP and going back 3 months (or going forward 9 months). For example, if the woman says that her LMP was on 10 January, her EDD will be 17 October. If a woman has cycles of 40 days, her revised EDD will be 29 October. In case she has short cycles of 22 days, her EDD will be 12 October.

In the event of some women having irregular cycles, varying from 28 days to 45 days to 60 days, it is worthwhile to enquire about the last to last menstrual period (LLMP).

History—The next step is to elicit a detailed obstetric history with regard to present pregnancy and the past ones (see Chapter 1).

PHYSICAL EXAMINATION

A thorough physical examination (including general, systemic and obstetric examination) is performed at the first visit. One must check for anemia and hypertension in particular.

The woman under discussion has presented with 2 months of amenorrhea. If her cycles are of 28–30 days and if she is pregnant, it is possible to confirm pregnancy clinically as the physical findings are characteristic (see Chapter 2).

LABORATORY INVESTIGATIONS

The following investigations are performed at the first visit:
1. Urine test for pregnancy if the clinical diagnosis is in doubt.
2. An ultrasound examination preferably transvaginal, if the period of gestation (POG) does not correspond to the period of amenorrhea
3. Estimation of hemoglobin
4. Urinalysis for sugar and albumin
5. Blood grouping and Rhesus typing if not done earlier or the woman has no record of it
6. VDRL for syphilis
7. Tests for hepatitis B and HIV (if necessary)

How does one decide whether a pregnant mother belongs to the high-risk category?

After the initial assessment, one needs to decide whether the woman under discussion is at risk of an adverse pregnancy outcome. In order to ensure effectiveness of ANC, a 'Risk approach' has been adopted. A pregnant woman can be formally evaluated against a checklist of risk factors. Whenever these risk factors are present, they influence obstetric decision making and outcome of pregnancy. The presence of any one or more of these factors must be considered as a risk to the mother and her fetus.

1.   Maternal characteristics   Age < 18 years or > 35 years
                                         Addiction to tobacco, alcohol, hard drugs

		Below poverty line (poor socioeconomic status)
2.	LMP details	LMP uncertain
		Oral pills 2 periods prior to LMP
		Cycle length > 30 days
		Vaginal bleeding since pregnancy
3.	Past obstetric history	Parity ≥ 5
		Congenital malformation
		Abortion (spontaneous or induced)
		Preterm labour
		Intruterine growth restriction (IUGR) or large baby
		Perinatal death
		Cesarean section or cervical suture
		Hypertension or eclampsia
		Third stage complications
4.	Medical history	Diabetes mellitus, cardiac or renal disease, thromboembolism
		Epilepsy
		Bronchial asthma, tuberculosis
5.	Family history	Diabetes mellitus
		Hypertension, pre-eclampsia or eclampsia in mother or sister
		Multiple pregnancy
		Congenital malformation
6.	Examination at first visit	Maternal weight < 45 kg or > 85 kg
		OR
		BMI < 18.5 or BMI > 30
		Maternal height 140 cm
		Blood pressure ≥ 140/90 mmHg
		Moderate to severe anemia
		Detection of cardiac murmur
		Uterus not corresponding to POG
		Gynecological disorder
		Rhesus negative

Once the pregnant mother is assessed thoroughly at the first visit, she is advised to return for regular ANC.

 What should be the schedule for subsequent antenatal visits?

The timing of subsequent visits is scheduled according to the POG and the presence of any complications. If all the parameters are within normal limits, traditionally the visits are scheduled at intervals of 4 weeks till 28 weeks and then every 2 weeks till 36 weeks and weekly thereafter. Fewer visits have been advocated when the pregnancy is uncomplicated or in circumstances where the pregnant woman or her relatives are educated and have easy access to a health care facility. If a woman is seen at 6 weeks of gestation, she may make her next visit at about 18 weeks.

In India, antenatal services are not accessible to the population residing in rural and urban slum areas; the minimum recommended number of visits is four. The first visit should be at 12–16 weeks of gestation, followed by the next one in the second trimester, the third visit at 28–32 weeks and the last one at 36–38 weeks.

 ## What should one do at each visit?

At each visit the mother should be asked if she has any bleeding/discharge per vaginum or abdominal pain, or any other complaints. The results of the investigations given at the earlier visit, if not already reviewed should be reviewed and appropriate advice given.

It is imperative to check:

❖ Weight
❖ Blood pressure (BP)
❖ Urine analysis
❖ Hemoglobin (Hb)
❖ Uterine fundal height
❖ Presentation and position of the fetus
❖ Fetal heart sounds

Weight—The average weight gain from the second trimester onwards should be 300–500 grams per week. An increase of less than 300 grams points to conditions like IUGR or maternal malnutrition. An excessive gain of 1000 grams per week must make one think of pre-eclampsia, multiple pregnancy or fetal macrosomia.

Blood pressure—If the BP is 140/90 mm Hg or more, it should be checked again after 6 hours. Alternatively, the woman may be requested to take rest for a while after which the BP is checked again. If two recordings of BP measure higher than or equal to 140/90 mm Hg after 20 weeks of gestation, a diagnosis of pregnancy induced hypertension (PIH) is made. The hypertension is said to be **pre-existing** when noted before 20 weeks of gestation.

Urine analysis—This is performed to detect sugar and albumin. The threshold for glucose is lowered and urine may test positive for sugar; under the circumstances, the blood glucose level must be estimated. The presence of albumin more than 1+ (300 mg in 24 hours) is pathological and is a pointer for further investigation.

Hemoglobin—The pregnant mother is said to be anemic if the level of hemoglobin is less than 11 g/dl (WHO 1989). According to the national recommendations, anemia is designated as moderate and severe respectively if the hemoglobin is 8 g/dl and 5 g/dl. Appropriate intervention should be planned according to the severity of the anemia.

Uterine fundal height—This is a useful parameter to assess the progress of pregnancy. Serial measurements of symphysiofundal height measured in centimetres plotted graphically (gravidogram) are useful in screening for fetal growth restriction; they could also be indicative of macrosomia, multiple pregnancy or polyhydramnios (see Chapter 3).

Presentation and position of the fetus—These are relevant after 34–36 weeks of pregnancy (see Chapter 3).

Fetal heart sounds—They reflect fetal wellbeing or otherwise (see Chapter 3).

 What other examination or investigations should be done?

An ultrasound examination is advised early in the first trimester if there is difficulty in assessing the POG. It is **mandatory** at 18–20 weeks in order to screen for congenital anomalies.

At 24–28 weeks the woman should be screened for diabetes mellitus if she:

❖ Has family history
❖ Is overweight
❖ Has given birth to large babies
❖ Has given birth to malformed babies
❖ Has recurrent pregnancy loss or vaginal infections

At 36–38 weeks one must look for any abnormal presentation and position and contracted pelvis. An examination to detect cephalopelvic disproportion is performed at 38 weeks. At this stage, one must plan the mode and place of delivery and refer the pregnant woman to an appropriate health facility if necessary.

 What advice should be given to the pregnant mother?

Schedule of antenatal visits—The pregnant woman must be explained about the need for regular ANC and must be given the date for the next visit depending on her health status and that of her fetus.

Nutrition—There is an increased nutritional demand during pregnancy. The pregnant woman should be advised to consume about 2800 Kcal/day, including 100 grams of proteins, 1500 mg of calcium, 70 mg of iron and 1 mg of folic acid. One must suggest food items rich in these elements, keeping affordability in mind. For example green leafy vegetables are rich in iron and folic acid; cereals like 'ragi' are rich in calcium.

Iron and Folic Acid—Iron is supplemented as tablets containing 60 mg of elemental iron, along with 0.5 mg of folic acid (IFA). The national recommendation is to supply 100 such tablets during pregnancy. In order to improve compliance, the woman must be counselled with reference to:

* Benefits of taking iron tablets
* Time of ingestion: 15 minutes after food
* Take a citrus fruit after food, as this increases the absorption of iron
* Reassurance about the black colour of her stools

Folic acid in a dose of 5 mg is advocated from prior to conception to 12 weeks of pregnancy in order to reduce the risk of neural tube malformations.

Breast feeding—At the first visit one must examine the breasts and advise correction of flat/retracted nipples if present. The woman must be counseled regarding the benefits of breast feeding during the antenatal visits so that she is well prepared to feed the baby.

Contraception—A dialogue regarding contraception should be initiated in order to bring about awareness of different methods available.

Clothing and footwear—The pregnant woman must be informed about the benefits of loose and comfortable clothing. She must be advised to use flat footwear and avoid high heels.

Immunisation against tetanus—In India one comes across cases of neonatal tetanus as a majority of deliveries take place at home under unhygienic conditions. According to the national immunisation schedule every pregnant mother must be administered an injection of tetanus toxoid 0.5 ml intramuscularly around 20 weeks of gestation and a second dose four to six weeks later. However, the second dose must be given at least four weeks before delivery in order to ensure protection of the newborn. Reinoculation is recommended every three years; if two doses were received less than three years earlier, a single booster dose is recommended.

Addictions—These must be enquired into. The commonest addiction is to tobacco, either in the form of smoking, chewing or snuff. Tobacco has a proven link with fetal growth restriction. The pregnant woman should be advised to stop it or to reduce it considerably. She must also be informed about the adverse effects of alcohol and hard drugs.

Drugs—The most common drugs pregnant women consume are vitamins, analgesics and antipyretics. Should there be a need for any others, one must select a drug that is relatively safe for the mother and her fetus.

Travel—This is best avoided in early and late stages of pregnancy. A woman with previous history of obstetric mishaps and complications in the current pregnancy should be advised against travel. A pregnant woman is often anxious about the effect of air travel on the fetus; she must be reassured that it is safe to travel since the cabin is pressurised.

Physical activity—This should not be restricted unless there is past history of spontaneous abortion or preterm delivery or complications in the present pregnancy.

Coitus—This is to be avoided if there is a threat of abortion or preterm delivery. In healthy pregnant women sexual intercourse is perfectly acceptable except in the last 4 weeks of pregnancy.

What are the minor complaints that a pregnant woman is likely to have?

A pregnant mother may present with some minor complaints that need attention.

Nausea and vomiting—These are common symptoms in early pregnancy. In most women proper dietary advice and reassurance are effective. Some of them may require antiemetics like doxylamine succinate at a dose of 10 mg at night, occasionally. Rarely, the vomiting can be quite severe and will need more aggressive management (see Chapter 5).

Heartburn—This is due to reflux of gastric contents into the esophagus, caused by relaxation of the sphincter at the lower end. The woman should be advised to take small frequent meals and avoid lying down flat after a meal. Antacids are prescribed if there is no relief .

Constipation—It occurs because of a raised level of progesterones, which slow down the transit time, and pressure of the enlarged uterus. The pregnant mother should be advised to take plenty of fluids, fruits and vegetables and daily exercise. If necessary mild laxatives and stool softeners may be prescribed. These measures will prevent the occurrence or worsening of anal fissures and hemorrhoids.

Pica—This is the craving for unusual food during pregnancy. Most pregnant women crave for pickles, but a few may consume excess of starch leading to iron deficiency anemia.

Ptyalism—This refers to excess salivation. No definite reason is attributed; it could be stimulated by excessive consumption of starch. The pregnant mother should be reassured if it is bothersome.

Backache—This is experienced by more than fifty per cent of women during pregnancy. It is caused by relaxation of the ligaments and lordosis. The woman should be advised regarding corrective posture and proper footwear. She should use a pillow to support her back, and should squat to pick up objects instead of bending. Application of local heat and analgesics are useful. However, if backache is persistent or there is a definite tenderness at any vertebral level, the woman must be referred to an orthopedic surgeon for further management.

Headache—This is a common complaint; if it is persistent in spite of symptomatic treatment, one must check for other causes like refractive errors. In the presence of hypertension, headache is associated with severe pre-eclampsia and imminent eclampsia.

Fatigue—This occurs most frequently in early pregnancy. The pregnant woman tends to feel sleepy which could be attributed to high levels of progesterone. The symptom could also be due to anemia, vomiting in early pregnancy and mechanical factors later on in pregnancy.

Varicosities of lower limbs may manifest during pregnancy; they could worsen if they pre-existed. The symptoms may vary from mild to severe discomfort after long hours of standing. Treatment consists of rest, elevation of legs and elastic stockings. Surgical intervention is not advised during pregnancy.

Leukorrhea—Pregnant women often complain of white discharge. It is mostly due to increased secretion of mucus from the cervix and transudation from the vagina due to increased levels of estrogens. The woman should be reassured.

If the discharge is greenish yellow and frothy, it could be due to trichmonal vaginitis. In case of bacterial vaginosis the discharge has a fishy odour. White discharge that is curd-like could be candidiasis. The woman should be treated appropriately, and with great caution in the first trimester of pregnancy.

 How should one plan for delivery?

The plan for delivery is dictated by the preexistence of risk factors or those that arise during pregnancy. The decision should be made with reference to the following points:

✤ POG at which the pregnancy should be terminated
✤ The method of delivery

❖ The type of health facility where delivery should take place

Therefore during the antenatal care, one should be vigilant and refer pregnant mothers to a carefully selected health facility. A pragmatic approach is to consider the following categories of mothers for delivery at home or at health centres where facilities for specialist care are not available:

❖ Absence of medical/surgical and gynecological disorders

❖ Normal obstetric history

❖ Gravidity second to fourth

❖ Normal fetal growth

❖ Normal fetopelvic relation (vertex presentation)

The need to ensure the presence of a skilled attendant is absolutely essential. This is the guideline issued by the Ministry of Health and Family Welfare and should be implemented in totality.

Key points

1. Antenatal care is a comprehensive systematic health care programme for pregnant mothers.

2. Preconception care improves both maternal and fetal outcome.

3. Efforts must be made to identify obstetric, gynecologic, medical and surgical complications.

4. The important recommendations for acceptable ANC are: four antenatal visits, iron and folic acid prophylaxis, administration of tetanus toxoid and measures for early detection of pre-eclampsia.

5. If necessary, women with no risk factors, second to fourth gravidae with normal fetopelvic relation may be selected for delivery at home or primary health centre.

6. Women must be counselled regarding issues like, nutrition, drugs, breast feeding and contraception.

CHAPTER 5

Vomiting in pregnancy

P. REDDI RANI

Vomiting in the early weeks of pregnancy is common. It is usually mild and occurs once or twice in the morning; the quantity is small and seldom affects the health of the mother to be. Occasionally, however, the vomiting persists and increases in frequency, with the result that very little nourishment is retained and the patient loses weight. Excessive vomiting in pregnancy is referred to as *hyperemesis gravidarum.*

Objectives

At the end of this chapter, the reader should be able to

- ❑ Define hyperemesis gravidarum.
- ❑ Enumerate important causes of vomiting in pregnancy.
- ❑ Perform appropriate clinical examination.
- ❑ Select relevant investigations.
- ❑ Plan appropriate treatment.

CLINICAL SCENARIO

A 20-year-old primigravida with nine weeks of pregnancy presents with excessive vomiting.

HISTORY

 What questions should be asked to get more information related to excessive vomiting?

✤ One must enquire about the *frequency of vomiting*, whether it is associated with abdominal pain or burning sensation in the abdomen, and the type of vomitus—whether it is bilious or blood-stained.

✤ *Period of amenorrhea and gravidity* of the patient are important—Hyperemesis is common in the first pregnancy and is usually limited to early pregnancy (6–16 weeks).

Persistent vomiting continuing beyond 16 weeks of pregnancy should make one suspect other conditions related to pregnancy like hydatidiform mole, acute hydramnios and multiple pregnancy.

The possibility of associated medical, surgical and gynecological disorders should always be borne in mind (Table 5.1).

PHYSICAL EXAMINATION

While performing physical examination, particular attention should be paid to the general condition of the patient.

✤ Dehydration of variable degree, sunken eyes, dry and thickly coated tongue, dry and inelastic skin and smell of acetone in the breath are observed in *severe hyperemesis.*

✤ When hyperemesis is not treated in the early stages, besides fluid–electrolyte imbalance and acidosis, jaundice and neurological manifestations like squint or nystagmus are likely to set in.

Table 5.1 Associated disorders

Medical	Surgical	Gynecological
Worm infestations	Acute appendicitis	Twisted ovarian tumour
Urinary tract infections	Peptic ulcer	Red degeneration of fibroid
Hepatitis	Intestinal obstruction	
Diabetic ketoacidosis	Cholecystitis	
Uremia		
Hiatus hernia		

❖ *Abdominal and vaginal examination* will help to confirm an early normal pregnancy and rule out the presence of disorders discussed earlier.

INVESTIGATIONS

The essential investigations that need to be performed are *urinalysis* and *biochemical investigations.*
❖ Urine output is decreased, concentrated with high specific gravity and with presence of acetone, diminished or absent chloride due to dehydration and ketosis.
❖ There is usually electrolyte imbalance due to excessive vomiting. Loss of water and salts in the vomitus, results in loss of plasma sodium, potassium and chloride resulting in hyponatremia and hypokalemia.
❖ Starvation results in acidosis and ketosis with hypoglycemia.

COMPLICATIONS

Complications in severe cases include neurologic complications like Wernicke's encephalopathy, peripheral neuritis and Korsakoff psychosis, and others like stress ulcer in stomach and jaundice.

MANAGEMENT

 What are the principles of management?
❖ In mild to moderate cases, reassurance and simple dietary regulations will suffice. The patient is advised to take small, frequent feeds; fatty foods should be avoided. Foods largely composed of carbohydrates, fruits, vegetables, dry toast, biscuits, jam and jelly are recommended. It is pragmatic to advise the patient to 'take the food she feels like taking'. Most patients show improvement with the above regimen. In some cases, it may be necessary to prescribe antiemetics. The patient must be advised to take doxylamine succinate 10 mg once in 24 hours. If vomiting persists, she may take upto three tablets in a day. Pyridoxine hydrochloride (vitamin B6) is safe and has been found to reduce nausea and vomiting.
❖ In severe cases, hospitalisation, correction of fluid, electrolyte and metabolic disturbances must be resorted to immediately. Pulse is recorded every four hours

and the blood pressure twice daily. The urine is checked twice daily for acetone, bile, sugar and specific gravity. Plasma electrolytes are measured and low potassium or sodium corrected by intravenous therapy. The intake and output of fluids are measured carefully in order to ensure a positive balance. Dehydration and ketosis are corrected by an intravenous infusion of 1 litre of 5% dextrose followed by one litre of Ringer lactate solution. Over a 24-hour period, the patient should receive 3–4 litres of fluids.

❖ Antiemetics like metoclopramide 10 mg intramuscularly twice or thrice daily, are effective in controlling vomiting.

❖ Easily assimilable carbohydrates in the form of glucose must be supplied in sufficient quantities to replace the depleted glycogen store and to correct acidosis.

❖ These measures help in the prevention of serious complications.

 ### Is there a place for termination of pregnancy in these women?

It may be necessary in the following situations:

❖ Steady deterioration in spite of therapy

❖ Pyrexia, hypotension, tachycardia

❖ Gradually increasing oliguria and proteinuria

❖ Appearance of jaundice

❖ Appearance of neurological complications

Hyperemesis gravidarum is a rare condition. Early admission along with prompt and effective therapy will prevent severe forms and the complications that arise therein.

Key points

1. Vomiting in early pregnancy is quite common and can be controlled with dietary adjustment and reassurance.

2. Excessive vomiting resulting in the deteriorating health of the pregnant woman is called hyperemesis gravidarum and requires hospitalisation.

3. Control of vomiting, correction of dehydration, electrolyte imbalance and ketosis, and administration of antiemetics are the main modes of treatment.

4. Effective treatment of mild and moderate forms of vomiting in pregnancy can prevent it from becoming severe.

CHAPTER 6

Vaginal bleeding in early pregnancy

P. REDDI RANI

Bleeding in early pregnancy is a common obstetric problem and is due to abortions in 95 per cent of cases. Two other important causes are ectopic pregnancy and vesicular mole. If missed, the bleeding may lead to life-threatening complications. Rarely, it may be due to implantation bleeding, lesions like polyp, cervical erosion, or cancer cervix co-existing with pregnancy.

Objectives

At the end of this chapter, the reader should be able to

❑ Enumerate and define the important causes of bleeding in early pregnancy.
❑ Distinguish between various types of abortions.
❑ Clinically differentiate abortion from vesicular mole.
❑ Select appropriate investigations to confirm the diagnosis.
❑ Plan the management.

CLINICAL SCENARIO

A 25-year-old primigravida with two months of amenorrhea presents with bleeding per vaginum and abdominal pain.

HISTORY

 What questions should be asked to get more information regarding symptoms with which the patient has presented?

Gestational age—Whenever a woman of reproductive age group presents with amenorrhea, one should always consider pregnancy, unless proved otherwise. The period of amenorrhea could be variable, but should not exceed 28 weeks, the period of viability. In India, expulsion of products of conception before 28 weeks of gestation is termed as abortion. The period of amenorrhea is very short or even absent in case of pregnancy in the fallopian tube (see Chapter 33).

In the patient under discussion, the period of gestation is two months; about 80 per cent of spontaneous abortions occur within the first 12 weeks of gestation.

Bleeding per vaginum—If the bleeding is persistent and the colour of blood is very dark, the patient has probably had a missed abortion. Fresh bleeding is suggestive of either threatened, incomplete or inevitable abortion. Bleeding is excessive in inevitable abortion and in some cases of incomplete abortion. Very scanty bleeding is characteristic of ectopic pregnancy and blood-stained serous discharge is associated with vesicular mole. Rarely, there is history of passing 'grape-like' vesicles.

Pain—The patient is most likely to complain of colicky pain in the lower abdomen. Its severity is maximum in an inevitable abortion. Acute pain is encountered in cases of disturbed ectopic pregnancy.

PHYSICAL EXAMINATION

1. **Pallor and tachycardia** are directly proportional to the amount of blood loss; as also the hypotension. Fever is generally absent, unless the partly retained products of conception are infected.
2. **Examination** of the breasts is useful if there are changes suggestive of pregnancy.
3. **Abdominal palpation**—Uterine enlargement of 14 weeks or more can be appreciated. Tenderness and guarding are usually absent, unless there is peritonitis. The uterus is bigger than warranted by the period of amenorrhea in 60 per cent, and feels 'doughy' in vesicular mole.
4. **Vaginal speculum examination** must be performed. Bluish discolouration of the cervix indicates pregnancy. This examination also helps to detect bleeding from the os and lesions on the cervix and the vagina.

5. **Bimanual examination**—A soft cervix is suggestive of pregnancy. The cervical os is closed in case of threatened abortion (Fig. 6.1) and open in inevitable and incomplete abortions (Fig. 6.2). It is important to note that the size of the uterus corresponds to the period of amenorrhea in case of threatened and inevitable abortion; in incomplete and missed abortions, the uterus is smaller than the period of gestation. The os is closed in case of missed abortion.

The clinical findings are summarised in Table 6.1 and are useful in arriving at a diagnosis.

Table 6.1 Findings in abortions

Type of abortion	Uterine size	Cervical os	Bleeding
Threatened	Corresponds to amenorrhea	Closed	Minimal
Inevitable	Corresponds to amenorrhea	Open; products felt.	Moderate to excessive
Incomplete	Smaller	Os open	Moderate to excessive
Missed	Smaller. Uterus feels firm.	Os closed	Dark, altered blood
Vesicular mole	Usually larger than period of gestation. Doughy consistency of uterus	Closed/open	Blood-stained serous discharge. Bleeding could be excessive during expulsion.

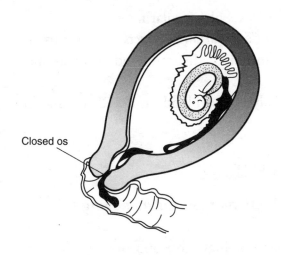

Fig. 6.1 Threatened abortion

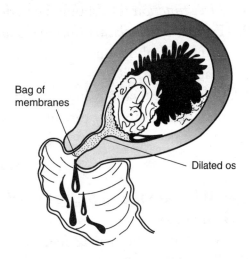

Fig. 6.2 Inevitable abortion

A patient with ectopic pregnancy also presents with the symptom triad of amenorrhea, pain in abdomen and bleeding per vaginum. As compared to disturbed intrauterine pregnancy, the pain is more severe and bleeding scanty. On vaginal examination, the movements of the cervix are excruciatingly tender, the uterus is usually enlarged upto eight weeks size of pregnancy and there may be a tender boggy mass in one of the fornices.

6. **Ultrasonography** is a useful investigation:

❖ Threatened abortion: In such a case, the fetus is alive and the process of expulsion has not yet begun. Ultrasonography is useful for detecting a live fetus and also for ruling out fetal malformation. This investigation must be performed before instituting conservative treatment for threatened abortion.

❖ Missed abortion: This term means that the fetus dies and the products are retained in the uterus. This finding should be confirmed ultrasonologically before advising evacuation of the uterus.

❖ **Unsafe abortion**—The other terms used are 'septic abortion' or 'illegal abortion'. It is important to remember that when an abortion is induced by an unskilled person, the chances of infection and trauma are very high. Ultrasonography helps to detect collection of pus in the pouch of Douglas or a tuboovarian mass.

7. **Pregnancy test** is a useful investigation to confirm pregnancy, but it could be positive for a while after fetal death. In cases of gestational trophoblastic diseases, it is positive in dilutions, but a quantitative serum estimation of β hCG is a better test.

8. *Liver function tests* should be performed in cases of vesicular mole.

9. Estimation of *plasma fibrinogen and fibrin degradation products* (FDP) is useful in missed abortion because of the likelihood of disseminated intravascular coagulation (DIC).

10. Other investigations like hemogram, urinalysis and blood group Rh typing are performed as for any case of hemorrhage.

MANAGEMENT

 What are the steps that need to be implemented for managing this patient?

The priority in the management of incomplete or inevitable abortions is to arrest bleeding. The steps are:

❖ Start IV line with a wide bore cannula (18 G).

❖ Administer sedation.

❖ Perform an evacuation, either suction or instrumental.

❖ Administer IV/IM ergometrine.

The priority in the management of vesicular mole and missed abortion is also uterine evacuation. However large a uterus is, in a case of vesicular mole, suction evacuation can be safely performed. In missed abortion, one has to choose an appropriate method depending on the size of the uterus. Dilatation and instrumental evacuation is feasible if the uterus is smaller than 14 weeks' size. Prostaglandins or extraamniotic instillation of ethacridine lactate have been advocated when the uterus is larger.

Hemorrhage, infection, DIC, renal failure and shock (both hemorrhagic and endotoxic) are significant complications of abortions.

Key points

1. Most causes of bleeding in early pregnancy can be diagnosed clinically.
2. Ultrasonography and estimation of β hCG are useful tools for evaluation and follow up.
3. Conservative treatment is instituted in case of threatened abortion only after confirming a live, normal fetus.
4. Immediate uterine evacuation is indicated in inevitable, incomplete abortion and in vesicular mole where bleeding could be profuse.
5. Strict adherence to aseptic and antiseptic precautions and correct estimation of the size and direction of uterus are essential in order to prevent infection and perforation of the uterus.

CHAPTER 7

Recurrent pregnancy loss

S. SOUNDARA RAGHAVAN

Inability or failure to conceive affects about 10 per cent of couples. Another group suffers from a more vexing problem of achieving pregnancy which repeatedly ends unsuccessfully. It may be difficult to identify a condition that is repeatedly responsible for failure of successive pregnancies. Some causes may not be treatable. However, it is worthwhile to investigate these patients so that the treatable conditions can be identified. In other situations, the information thus gained can be used to counsel the couple regarding the prognosis.

Objectives

At the end of this chapter, the reader should be able to

- ❑ Define recurrent pregnancy loss.
- ❑ Elicit relevant history from a woman presenting with recurrent pregnancy loss.
- ❑ Perform appropriate clinical examination.
- ❑ Select relevant investigations.
- ❑ Suggest appropriate treatment.
- ❑ Prognosticate and counsel couples who have had recurrent pregnancy loss.

CLINICAL SCENARIO

A 27-year-old woman, pregnant for the third time, presents with 11 weeks' pregnancy. She has previously had an abortion at the 9th week of pregnancy and another abortion at the 12th week of pregnancy.

Can this woman be considered to have had recurrent pregnancy loss?
Pregnancy loss may occur after the period of viability, preterm delivery, intrauterine death, fetal anomalies or earlier as abortion. It may also include preclinical postconceptional loss. Pregnancy loss is usually defined as recurrent (RPL), if there are three or more consecutive pregnancy losses. Often, the term is used as equivalent to recurrent abortions. This is because the majority of RPL are recurrent abortions. Whatever the nature of pregnancy loss, it is important to ascertain whether there is a cause which repeatedly operates and if it has an influence on her future reproductive career. In that strict theoretical sense, the patient mentioned above may not come under the category of RPL. However, even a single pregnancy loss may upset the woman to such an extent that she seeks medical help. Hence, it may be necessary to give attention to women with one or two pregnancy losses also.

HISTORY

Eliciting history in the above patient

1. It is important to note the *age* of both the husband and wife. Increased maternal and paternal age increases the risk of abortion.
2. *Parity* is also important as the risk of abortion increases with increasing parity.
3. Any history of *bleeding or abdominal pain* in the current pregnancy should be enquired into.
4. The *menstrual history* of oligo- or hypomenorrhea may suggest problems like polycystic ovarian syndrome (PCOS), luteal phase defects (LPD) and progesterone deficiency.
5. Detailed enquiry should be made about the previous pregnancies. The risk of pregnancy loss increases with each *previous pregnancy* loss. A woman who has had three abortions in the past is likely to lose nearly half her pregnancies.
6. The *duration of gestation* at which the earlier pregnancy losses occurred should be noted.
7. One must enquire whether the marriage is *consanguineous* or not.

The majority of early abortions are due to genetic abnormalities, endocrine defects and immunological causes, in that order.

Abortions occurring later in the pregnancy may be due to anatomical defects like cervical incompetence and infections like syphilis. The history in cervical incompetence is typically painless expulsion of products in mid-trimester, preceded by glairy mucus or rupture of membranes. The fetus may be expelled alive.

 ### What are the significant points in the past history, which may be useful in RPL?

If the mother has been diagnosed to have diabetes, hypertension, thyroid disorders, infections like toxoplasma, cytomegalovirus and chronic urinary infections or other renal diseases, there may be an increased risk of RPL. History of treatment with certain drugs like antimetabolites may also be important.

 ### Is family history relevant?

History of chromosomal disorders in the family and presence of diseases like diabetes in the previous generation may be important. If the mother of the patient had been exposed to diethyl stilboesterol (DES) when she was carrying the patient, the patient may have a small T shaped uterus or cervical incompetence.

 ### Does the personal behaviour of the woman or her partner influence pregnancy outcome?

Smoking and use of alcohol and hard drugs can all predispose to pregnancy loss. Sexually transmitted diseases like syphilis, chlamydia, ureaplasma and mycoplasma infections can also cause pregnancy loss. There is some evidence to suggest that excess sexual activity, particularly during pregnancy, may lead to pregnancy loss in susceptible women.

EXAMINATION

A thorough general examination should include recording of blood pressure, looking for lymphadenopathy, evidence of renal disease like edema, examination of the neck for thyroid gland and features of hypothyroidism like coarse skin, hoarse voice, slow reflexes or findings suggestive of hyperthyroidism like tachycardia, prominent eyeballs or tremor. Presence of oily skin, acne, obesity and mild hirsutism may suggest PCOS with luteal defects. Any clinical feature suggestive of congenital disorder should be looked for. 'Butterfly rash' on the face may suggest SLE.

A pelvic examination may help to rule out anatomical defects in the genital tract. The status of the cervix is noted, and an open cervical os allowing easy passage of an

8 mm dilator in the nonpregnant state suggests cervical incompetence.

The uterus is bimanually palpated carefully. Its size, shape, position and mobility are noted. The presence of lesions like fibroids is looked for. Many of the anatomical defects may not be clinically detectable.

INVESTIGATIONS

Since investigations for RPL can be very tedious and expensive one has to choose investigations judiciously.

Apart from investigations to assess the general condition of the patient, a serological test for syphilis may be done. Pelvic ultrasonography is essential in all patients with RPL. This will help to diagnose an anembryonic pregnancy. It may also help in checking for anatomical abnormalities of the uterus, including cervical incompetence, presence of fibroids and polycystic ovaries. The last three conditions can be diagnosed in the nonpregnant state also. In addition, ultrasonography during pregnancy may help in prognosis and planning management.

Glucose tolerance test (GTT), thyroid function test, hysteroscopy or hystero-salpingography in the nonpregnant state and serum luteinising hormone levels may be checked as indicated. While GTT may be conducted as a routine, the other tests may be done if the first set of tests are negative. Serological tests searching for a cause include TORCH study, lupus anticoagulant (APTT, KCT), and antithrombin III deficiency. Anti-nuclear or anti-DNA antibodies will be found in SLE. ELISA testing for antiphospholipid antibodies can be done.

Karyotyping of the couple is an important investigation in RPL, particularly if the abortions have occurred in early pregnancy or there has been evidence of anembryonic pregnancy. If possible, the abortus can also be studied for chromosomal abnormalities.

MANAGEMENT

 What are the steps that need to be implemented for managing this patient?

In this case, treatment will depend on the cause. Infections, if detected, can usually be treated easily. Treatment of toxoplasmosis is expensive and prolonged. Spiramycin is used throughout pregnancy for treating toxoplasmosis.

If there is abnormal karyotype in the father, the risk has to be assessed in consultation with a geneticist. It may be necessary to resort to donor insemination. If the mother has abnormal karyotype, oocyte donation may be necessary along with assisted reproduction techniques (ART) . For couples who can accept adoption, it may be a better and less expensive alternative.

Endocrine abnormalities like diabetes, thyroid dysfunction, and PCOS should be appropriately treated. Luteal defects are treated with human chorionic gonadotrophin (hCG) and/or progestogens till about 14 weeks of pregnancy.

There is much controversy about treatment of autoimmune or alloimmune diseases. While it is easy to treat SLE with steroids, pregnancy in such a patient may be fraught with numerous complications. Similarly diabetes, hypertension and renal disease may make the course of pregnancy very difficult and the outcome may not be predictable. In the management of recurrent abortions due to antiphospholipid antibodies, prednisolone, aspirin, heparin and plasmapheresis have all been used with varying success.

Immunostimulation using paternal leucocytes, pooled donor cells or trophoblastic membrane has been reported to be successful for alloimmune aborters.

Surgical management

One group of women, who may benefit from surgical treatment is those with cervical incompetence. Cervical cerclage during pregnancy may be beneficial to this group. Various operations like Shirodkar cerclage, McDonald procedure and Wurm stitch are used. The outcome may be better when the operation is done prophylactically than when done therapeutically. However, some authors believe that there is no evidence to suggest that prophylactic cerclage is useful.

Other indications for surgical treatment may be correction of anatomical abnormalities of uterus, like excision of uterine septum and unification of bicornuate uterus in the nonpregnant state. Sometimes there may be associated cervical incompetence which may require attention.

There is not much evidence of myomectomy being beneficial in women with RPL; it should be the last resort.

PROGNOSIS AND COUNSELLING

Prognosis in the current pregnancy will depend on past history. Women who have had one loss tend to have higher risk of a subsequent loss. The risk of spontaneous abortion in a woman with no loss is about 15 per cent. It increases to 19 per cent after one abortion, 35 per cent after two and 47 per cent after three losses. The risk reduces if there has been one live child.

The prognosis will also depend on the cause of RPL. Infections seem to have better prognosis. Anatomical abnormalities may come next. Immunological conditions and chronic diseases like renal disease, diabetes, thyroid dysfunction will have varying outcome, generally not very good.

Prognosis for the present pregnancy will also depend on the findings of ultra-sonography, chorion villus sampling and karyotype. Abnormal parental karyotype may require extensive counselling for adoption or donor assisted reproduction techniques.

Key points

1. RPL is defined as three or more consecutive pregnancy losses and is usually due to recurrent abortions.
2. The majority of the early abortions are due to genetic abnormalities, endocrine defects and immunological causes. Later abortions may be due to cervical incompetence and infections like syphilis.
3. Cervical incompetence typically presents as recurrent, painless mid-trimester abortions preceded by glairy mucus or rupture of membranes. The cervix allows easy passage of an 8 mm dilator in the nonpregnant state and is treated by cerclage.
4. Pelvic ultrasonography is essential in all patients with RPL to diagnose anembryonic pregnancies, uterine abnormalities, fibroids and polycystic ovaries. It also helps to prognosticate and plan management.
5. Infections are usually treated easily. Spiramycin is used throughout pregnancy for toxoplasmosis.
6. Abnormal karyotype in parents may be treated with donor sperms/ova and assisted reproductive techniques. Alternatively, adoption may be considered.
7. Luteal phase defects are treated with hCG till about 14 weeks of pregnancy.

8.   Prednisolone, aspirin, heparin and plasmapheresis have all been used with varying success in patients with antiphospholipid antibodies.

9.   Surgical excision of uterine septum or unification of bicornuate uterus in the nonpregnant state may be useful in patients with uterine abnormalities. Associated cervical incompetence, if any, should also be treated.

10. The prognosis depends on the number of previous losses and the cause. The risk of spontaneous abortion is 15, 19, 35 and 47 per cent after 0, 1, 2 and 3 previous losses, but reduces if there has been one live child. Infections have a better prognosis followed by anatomical abnormalities. Results in patients with immunological conditions and chronic diseases are variable and often unsatisfactory.

CHAPTER 8

Breathlessness in pregnancy

GITA RAJAGOPALAN

The increased demand for oxygen in pregnancy is met by an increase in tidal volume and minute oxygen uptake in the lungs. Though there is no definite increase in the respiratory rate, there is an increased awareness of a desire to breathe, thought to be mediated by progesterone. However, breathlessness implies an element of distress due to the need for increased respiratory effort, accompanied by an increase in the respiratory rate. There are several causes for breathlessness, some of which are of a serious nature and require prompt attention.

Objectives

At the end of this chapter, the reader should be able to

- ❏ Enumerate causes of breathlessness in pregnancy.
- ❏ Perform relevant clinical examination.
- ❏ Choose appropriate investigations and interpret the results.
- ❏ Plan appropriate therapy.

CLINICAL SCENARIO

A 25-year-old primigravida at 32 weeks gestation presents at the emergency medical services department with a history of breathlessness of two days duration.

HISTORY

 What questions should be asked to acquire more information regarding the symptoms with which the patient has presented?

1. If the patient is acutely symptomatic, only a brief history is to be elicited. Her partner or relatives may also provide details.

2. It is necessary to elicit *history of previous episodes* and whether the patient is known to have *bronchial asthma* and being treated for the same. It would be relevant to enquire about history of a similar complaint in other family members.

3. One should enquire regarding information suggestive of *rheumatic fever* in the past. If there is such a history, one should ask if the patient is on treatment for rheumatic heart disease, which is quite common among the population from the lower socio-economic class.

4. About 40–80 per cent of pregnant women in India continue to be anemic and could be suffering from breathlessness. Therefore, it is important to ask whether the patient was taking hematinics during pregnancy. It is useful to find out what could be responsible for anemia; whether there was any history of blood loss like piles or heavy periods preceding pregnancy.

5. History of fever, cough with expectoration and hemoptysis in the past are suggestive of an *acute* or *chronic respiratory infection;* the possibility of tuberculosis should always be kept in mind.

6. Did the patient notice any sudden increase in abdominal distension recently? Overdistension due to acute polyhydramnios and multiple pregnancy can cause breathlessness by further splinting of the diaphragm.

7. Whether the patient has shown any signs of *psychiatric illness* at any time, should be ascertained.

CAUSES

The different causes for breathlessness in pregnancy (based on frequency of occurrence) are:

❖ Anemia
❖ Respiratory infections
❖ Bronchial asthma

- ❖ Heart disease
- ❖ Obstetric causes
- ❖ Hysterical hyperventilation
- ❖ Adult respiratory distress syndrome (ARDS)

GENERAL PHYSICAL EXAMINATION

The patient will appear very ill in case of a severe attack of bronchial asthma and cardiac failure consequent to either organic heart disease or severe anemia.

The respiratory rate, heart rate, blood pressure and temperature should be recorded. A note must be made about the presence of pallor, cyanosis and pedal edema.

SYSTEMIC EXAMINATION

1. *Cardiovascular system*—Evidence of organic heart disease, type of valvular lesions, cardiac failure, cardiomegaly and arrhythmias should be checked for.
2. *Respiratory system*—An examination must be performed to corroborate any evidence of bronchospasm like the presence of rhonchi. Presence of crepitations and rhonchi point to the possibility of respiratory infection. The presence of features suggestive of a cavity or pleural effusion indicate pulmonary tuberculosis.
3. *Obstetric examination*—An abdominal examination helps to establish a cause for the overdistension such as multifetal gestation where multiple fetal parts are felt with three or more fetal poles. Polyhydramnios is characterised by fluid thrill and difficulty in palpating fetal parts. Presence of tumour/ascites can also cause abdominal overdistension.
4. *A hysterical reaction* can be detected by the anxious and disturbed attitude of the patient and a tendency to exaggerate symptoms when being observed. ARDS is usually secondary to septicemia.

INVESTIGATIONS

1. Complete *hematological investigation* including peripheral blood smear is useful to assess the extent of anemia. Leukocytosis will occur in acute respiratory infection.
2. *Sputum* is subjected to Gram stain and culture. Staining for acid-fast bacilli must

be performed whenever there is history of contact, evening rise in temperature and cough with expectoration of long duration.

3. *X-ray of chest* is useful in the diagnosis of pulmonary tuberculosis.
4. *ECG* and *echocardiography* are required in case of cardiac disease.
5. *Pulmonary function tests* and *arterial blood gas analysis* are indicated in bronchial asthma.

MANAGEMENT

 How does one proceed to manage a patient with breathlessness?

Treatment depends on the cause of breathlessness. However, severe anemia, bronchial asthma and cardiac failure due to organic heart disease continue to be commonly encountered in obstetric practice in this country and *require immediate attention*.

1. General measures:
   * The patient must be admitted to the hospital.
   * She must be in a propped-up position.
   * Oxygen must be administered.
2. *Severe anemia* with hemoglobin level of less than 6 g/dl is treated with transfusion of blood or packed cells. Oral and parenteral iron therapy will take six weeks to be effective. Parenteral iron is mainly indicated when there is noncompliance or intolerance to oral iron therapy.

   Mild to *moderate anemia* is implied when hemoglobin level is less than 11 g/dl and more than 6 g/dl.
   * Oral iron 200 mg tds should be given.
   * If not tolerated, iron dextran complex 100 mg deep IM (gluteal) should be given after checking sensitivity.
   * Total dose of iron should be calculated according to patient's body weight and hemoglobin level.
3. *Management of cardiac failure*—The principles of management of cardiac failure are similar to that in the nonpregnant state. Digitalisation and diuretics along with bronchodilators, oxygen and sometimes morphine, are used. Cardiology and cardiothoracic surgery consultation should be sought whenever a valvular lesion is suspected. If there is no improvement with medical treatment, surgery such as mitral valvotomy or balloon valvuloplasty can be done in pregnancy.

Treatment of pulmonary edema/cardiac failure

- ❖ Propped-up position
- ❖ Oxygen by mask/tent
- ❖ Inj morphine 15 mg IM
- ❖ Inj frusemide 40 mg IV
- ❖ Parenteral bronchodilators (aminophylline IV) if required
- ❖ Tablet digoxin 0.5 mg followed by 0.25 mg daily

4. *Bronchial asthma*—The management will depend on the severity of attack. Status asthmaticus will require management in intensive care setup. Maintenance therapy with oral bronchodilators or inhaler therapy may be used in less severe cases.

   Treatment:

   A. Episodic attacks

   Tablet theophylline 100 mg tds

   Inhaler – sodium chromoglycate

   Tablet terbutaline 2.5–5 mg tds

   B. Status asthmaticus

   Blood gas analysis

   Ventilatory support

   Inj epinephrine 0.3–0.5 ml (1:1000 solution SC)

   Inj terbutaline 250 μg IM every 15 min x 3

   Inj hydrocortisone 250 mg IV 4–6 hourly

5. *Obstetric management*—There is usually no indication for inducing labour. Most patients go into labour spontaneously. Intensive monitoring of the mother and the fetus is important all through. The second stage should be cut short with outlet forceps or ventouse to avoid undue straining by the mother. In patients with severe anemia, adequate blood should be kept ready for use.

   Prophylactic administration of methylergometrine MUST be ensured to reduce blood loss in anemia. However, if the patient is suffering from a cardiac lesion, this drug should be withheld.

PREVENTION AND EARLY DETECTION

During the antenatal period, one must ensure adequate intake of iron and folic acid to prevent the occurrence of *anemia (defined as Hb <11 g per cent)*. Since about 40–80 per cent of antenatal mothers are anemic, they will require iron and folic acid in therapeutic doses. Hemoglobin level must be checked at the first visit and later as required. Any underlying cause for anemia, such as hookworm infestation, should be detected and treated.

In the case of a heart disease complicating pregnancy, a cardiology consultation may be obtained. All measures should be directed towards preventing cardiac failure and infective endocarditis. Prophylactic diuretics and digitalis, prevention of anemia, infections, admission at 28–30 weeks of pregnancy will help minimise complications. Unnecessary pelvic examination should be avoided. Bacterial endocarditis prophylaxis should be instituted during labour or before any other invasive procedure.

Key points

1. Breathlessness is a normal feature of pregnancy and does not necessarily represent cardiorespiratory disease.
2. In the absence of any other symptom, anemia is the commonest cause of dyspnea. It must be detected and treated, and measures must be taken to prevent it.
3. Other causes of breathlessness are bronchial asthma and rheumatic heart disease.
4. Immediate treatment should be instituted in case of acute asthma, cardiac failure due to severe anemia and heart disease. Patients should then be referred to institutions having facilities for intensive care.
5. Severity of the diseases and consequent maternal morbidity and mortality can be avoided by detecting and treating the diseases early in pregnancy.

CHAPTER 9

Fever during pregnancy

S. SOUNDARA RAGHAVAN

Fever is a fairly common problem. Though fever lasting for a few days may not worry the patient, its occurrence in pregnancy is likely to cause concern. The causes of fever may range from a simple viral fever to serious or potentially serious conditions. Fever due to urinary tract infection (UTI) is more common in pregnancy, but one should not overlook other causes of fever. When a patient reports with fever during pregnancy, the physician should remember the effect of fever itself as well as that of the disease that causes fever on pregnancy and the implications in pregnancy due to the possible treatment.

Objectives

At the end of this chapter, the reader should be able to

- ❑ Enumerate the common causes of fever during pregnancy.
- ❑ Elicit appropriate history from a pregnant woman who presents with fever.
- ❑ Perform clinical examination in order to detect the cause of fever.
- ❑ Choose relevant investigations.
- ❑ Select drugs rationally.
- ❑ Anticipate, diagnose and treat the possible effects of fever and the disease which causes the fever, on the outcome of pregnancy.

CLINICAL SCENARIO

A primigravida, married for six months and 12 weeks pregnant, presents with fever of five days duration and vomiting of one day duration.

It is important to remember that a large number of infectious diseases can cause fever during pregnancy. By far the most common cause of fever during pregnancy is urinary tract infection. Later in pregnancy, one must consider the possibility of chorioamnionitis following premature rupture of membranes (PROM). The occurrence of viral fever and respiratory infections including tuberculosis is fairly frequent. Filariasis and malaria are endemic to parts of India and must not be ruled out.

HISTORY

 What questions should be asked to gain more information regarding symptoms with which the patient has presented?

When a patient presents with fever, one should find out about the severity, type and time of fever.

Enquiry should be made about chills and rigors, headache, bodyache and pains. Viral fevers present with moderate (upto 39°C) intermittent fever associated with significant bodyache, malaise and headache. Presence of chills and rigors is associated with urinary infections and parasitic infections. Fever may be high (40°C) in these infections as also in conditions like enteric fever. Parasitic infections may be characterised by 'night sweats'.

Dysuria, urgency and frequency characterise cystitis and could accompany urethritis. There may also be suprapubic pain, pyuria and hematuria. Past history of treatment for UTI also contributes to diagnosis. Running nose, cough, sneezing and sore throat may suggest upper respiratory infection. History of loss of appetite, loss of weight, fever at night and history of contact should lead to the possibility of tuberculosis.

In a case of chorioamnionitis, the patient presents with history of rupture of membranes or watery or offensive discharge per vaginum and pain abdomen.

CLINICAL EXAMINATION

It is useful to record the temperature at 4 or 6 hour intervals and maintain a chart. This helps to study the pattern and severity of the fever.

Suffused eyes, rhinorrhea and congested throat indicate viral fever or upper respiratory infections. High temperature with lower abdominal or loin tenderness may suggest urinary infections, particularly acute pyelonephritis. One may detect hepatosplenomegaly in some patients with malaria or enteric fever; painful limb/leg swelling could be due to filarial lymphangitis. Uterine tenderness and discharge of infected amniotic fluid is diagnostic of chorioamnionitis.

Inadequate nourishment, presence of cervical lymph nodes, respiratory findings like crepitations and bronchial breathing favour a diagnosis of tuberculosis.

The importance of a complete general and systemic examination, with the help of a physician if necessary, to diagnose less common causes of fever, cannot be overemphasised.

INVESTIGATIONS

The basic investigation of fever during pregnancy includes estimation of hemoglobin, total and differential counts, and a study of peripheral smear for malarial or filarial parasites.

Examination of urine under the microscope for the presence of pus cells is useful to detect urinary infection. If there is a significant number of pus cells (5–10/HPF), the urine should be cultured with antibiogram to help in choosing the correct drug. Microscopic examination of the liquor amnii and its culture is useful if chorioamnionitis is suspected.

Radiological investigations should be kept to a minimum during pregnancy. However, if there is strong clinical suspicion of pulmonary tuberculosis, a skiagram of the chest with shielding of the uterus can be taken. A single exposure will not harm the fetus.

Further selection of investigations will depend upon the clinical situation. Microbiological examination of sputum, Widal and tests for autoimmune diseases may have to be done when required.

MANAGEMENT

 How does one proceed to manage this patient?

The principles of treatment of fever during pregnancy include control of fever, adequate hydration, antibiotic therapy when indicated, and monitoring of the condition of the mother and the fetus.

Paracetamol is an antipyretic with practically no side effects and no teratogenic effect. It may be given in doses of 500–1000 mg every 4–6 hours. Ibuprofen can be used where anti-inflammatory effect is desired, in doses of 400–1200 mg/day; this drug may produce gastritis.

Antibiotic therapy should be limited to urinary infections, proven bacterial respiratory infections, chorioamnionitis and infections like enteric fever. The choice of antibiotics should preferably be restricted to those antibiotics that do not cross the placental barrier. The tetracycline group of drugs and chloramphenicol are to be avoided; the safest drugs are penicillins and cephalosporins. Aminoglycosides should be used with caution. Amoxycillin, erythromycin, azithromycin and roxithromycin may be useful in respiratory and some urinary infections if the organisms are sensitive to these antibiotics. The treatment schedules for UTI, enteric fever and malaria are given below. Any one of the following antibiotic regimens may be used as indicated.

Treatment of urinary infection
1. Capsule ampicillin 500 mg 6 hourly x 7–10 days
2. Tablet cotrimoxazole 2 bd x 7–10 days (avoid in early and late pregnancy)
3. Tablet norfloxacin 400 mg bd x 7 days (avoid in early and late pregnancy)
4. Tablet nitrofurantoin 100 mg tds x 7 days (avoid in early and late pregnancy)
5. Inj. gentamicin 3–5 mg/kg/day in divided doses x 7–10 days; renal toxicity to be remembered
6. Inj. cefotaxime 1 g IV 8–12 hourly x 7 days; expensive; available only for parenteral use
7. The same regimen should be given for 3 days, if the urinary infection has occurred for the first time and is uncomplicated.

Treatment of enteric fever
1. Tablet ciprofloxacin 500 mg bd x 10–14 days
2. Tablet furazolidine 100 mg tid x 10–14 days
3. Capsule chloromycetin 500 mg 6 hourly x 10–14 days
4. Inj. ceftriaxone 1–2 g IV once/twice a day x 5 days

Benefits of antituberculous and antimalarial treatment outweigh the risks and can be used during pregnancy should the need arise. However, it should be remembered that when the mother is considerably ill, any drug might be used to treat her, in spite of the pregnancy.

Treatment of malaria

Tablet chloroquine	10 mg/kg stat
	5 mg/kg after 6 hours
	5 mg/kg in 2 divided doses x 2 days
Tablet metakelfen	2 tablets stat
Tablet primaquine	15 mg daily x 7 days
(falciparum infections)	

EFFECTS OF FEVER ON PREGNANCY

While mild fever may have no significant adverse effect on pregnancy, it is necessary to remember that there may be insensible fluid loss, which is greater during pregnancy. Adequate fluid intake should be ensured. This may also help in urinary tract infections.

Acute febrile episodes may cause death of the fetus leading to abortion, intrauterine death or preterm labour. It is essential to assess the fetal condition after the mother improves. Similarly, infections like malaria and some bacterial infections like chorioamnionitis may cause the death of the fetus or cause intrauterine fetal infections like congenital pneumonia.

Termination of pregnancy may have to be considered if fever is due to viral exanthemata in early pregnancy. Pregnancy termination will also be needed if the fever has caused fetal death.

Key points

1. Fever is a common symptom among pregnant mothers residing in the tropics.
2. During pregnancy, common causes of fever are urinary infections and viral fever.
3. Urinary tract infection or chorioamnionitis have a deleterious effect on the outcome of pregnancy.
4. The possibility of malaria, filariasis and enteric fever should be considered.
5. A pragmatic approach is advocated for the use of antipyretics and antibiotics during pregnancy.

CHAPTER 10

Abdominal pain during pregnancy

S. SOUNDARA RAGHAVAN

Abdominal pain is perhaps one of the commonest symptoms during pregnancy and it causes considerable anxiety. Abdominal pain may be due to a variety of conditions ranging from the mild pain of normal pregnancy caused by uterine distension, displacement and pressure on adjacent structures, peritoneal stretching or 'round ligament spasm', to the severe pain caused by dangerous abruptio placentae or acute surgical conditions. Therefore, the tendency on the part of the physician to dismiss the pain as a part of the minor disturbances of normal pregnancy is not an acceptable attitude. Every attempt should be made to exclude serious conditions by a thorough history-taking and clinical examination, before reassuring the patient about the innocuous nature of the pain.

Objectives

At the end of this chapter, the reader should be able to

- ❑ Enumerate the causes of abdominal pain during pregnancy.
- ❑ Obtain necessary information from a patient presenting with abdominal pain during pregnancy.
- ❑ Perform a thorough clinical examination.
- ❑ Choose the necessary investigations.
- ❑ Detect provisionally the cause of abdominal pain during pregnancy.
- ❑ Plan appropriate treatment keeping in mind the pregnant condition, the duration of pregnancy and fetal well-being.

CLINICAL SCENARIO

A second gravida presents at 24 weeks of pregnancy with abdominal pain of 2 days' duration and vomiting.

HISTORY

 ### How should one proceed to take a relevant history?

It is necessary to get details of the pain—its onset, type, duration, severity, radiation and whether it is continuous or intermittent.

Abdominal pain due to the so-called minor disturbances of pregnancy is usually mild, nondescript, insidious in onset and does not persist for long. On the other hand, if the onset is acute, the pain is severe, persists for a considerable time and radiates, it could be caused by a serious condition. Such pain is usually associated with other symptoms.

Pain of a burning nature related to food intake in most cases is due to gastro-esophageal reflux which is related to a reduced 'barrier' pressure (difference between gastric and lower esophageal sphincter pressure). This distressing symptom commonly starts in the third trimester but could also commence in early pregnancy. Severe epigastric pain is experienced by patients suffering from severe pre-eclampsia/imminent eclampsia and it is due to stretching of the liver capsule.

Constipation is common during pregnancy due to reduced gut motility and pressure of the enlarged uterus. It is associated with vague abdominal pain.

 ### What are the other symptoms about which one should enquire?

Pain caused by obstetric conditions may be associated with either vaginal bleeding or discharge. The patient may be able to appreciate hardening of the uterus with the intermittent colicky pain. The pain usually radiates to the lower abdomen and the medial aspect of thighs.

Nausea and vomiting can be associated with severe pain due to any cause, but the presence of these symptoms may also occur in urinary infection or in surgical conditions like appendicitis. Severe intractable vomiting is found in conditions like intestinal obstruction. Hematemesis with pain may be due to peptic ulcer disease. Occurrence of fever usually indicates an infection, commonly urinary; these patients may also suffer from dysuria and chills and rigors.

Symptoms like diarrhea, and tenesmus are found in amebiasis, shigellosis or salmonellosis. Constipation when absolute, suggests an intestinal obstruction. Yellow urine with abdominal pain may suggest hepatitis, cholecystitis, or rarely pancreatitis. If there is hematuria, calculous urinary disease has to be considered. Tea-coloured urine may indicate porphyria. Occasionally, pneumonia may present with abdominal pain.

An enquiry should be made about a history of interference with pregnancy which may not be easily forthcoming.

 What is the importance of menstrual history?

If the history of amenorrhea is short and there is abdominal pain, one has to consider abortion which is usually associated with vaginal bleeding. It is important to remember that ectopic pregnancy often presents as abdominal uneasiness, pain, diarrhea and irregular vaginal bleeding; amenorrhea may or may not be present. Very severe pain associated with vomiting points to 'acute abdomen'; if it is confined to lower abdomen, one must proceed as indicated in Chapter 33. Abruptio placentae should be considered if the period of amenorrhea is 28 weeks or more.

With good history-taking, it is usually possible to guess at, if not actually identify, the probable causes of abdominal pain.

GENERAL EXAMINATION

The general condition of the patient should be assessed by recording pulse, blood pressure and temperature. The degree of pallor should be noted. The patient is likely to be in a state of shock in acute conditions and will also be pale in hemorrhagic conditions. There may be significant dehydration and acidotic breathing. One may also find profuse sweating and air hunger.

Assessment of the general condition and steps to correct abnormalities are important and may be life-saving. Some measures may be started even before the diagnosis is established.

 What are the difficulties in eliciting findings in a patient with abdominal pain in pregnancy?

Till the end of the first trimester, it may be possible to appreciate the abdominal findings in a patient with pregnancy, just as in the nonpregnant condition. In the later stages of pregnancy, the enlarging uterus makes it more difficult to identify signs like exact location of tenderness (like McBurney's point in appendicitis), presence of a mass, thickened colon and cecal gurgle. Other signs suggesting peritoneal irritation like guarding and rigidity may be difficult to appreciate, and may be mistaken for a rigid uterus. Free fluid, if present in small to moderate quantities, may be missed. It may even be difficult to appreciate bowel sounds. Percussion of the abdomen is often not performed during pregnancy, but could be useful in suspected cases of intestinal obstruction.

 Is there any way of clinically differentiating the pain caused by uterine or adnexal condition from that caused by extragenital disease?

With the patient in supine position, the abdomen is palpated and the point of tenderness is located. With the examining hand still in position, she is turned to the left lateral position. If the pain shifts to the left, the pain is likely to be due to a uterine or adnexal cause. If there is no change, the cause of pain could be outside the genital tract. This is known as *Alder sign.*

CAUSES OF ABDOMINAL PAIN DURING PREGNANCY

Obstetric causes

Early pregnancy
Abortion including induced abortion
Ectopic pregnancy
Cystitis
Acute retention of urine

Late pregnancy
Labour pains
Severe pre-eclampsia
Abruptio placentae
Rupture uterus
Torsion of gravid uterus

Urinary infections including pyelonephritis can occur at any stage in pregnancy.

Surgical causes

Appendicitis
Intestinal obstruction

	Cholecystitis, gall stones
	Calculous urinary disease
	Pancreatitis
Gynecological causes	Torsion of ovarian cyst
	Red degeneration of fibroid uterus
Medical causes	Colitis
	Peptic ulcer
	Diarrhea, dysentery

A vaginal speculum examination must be performed to detect bleeding/discharge from the cervical canal. A bimanual examination is essential to detect cervical dilatation if the patient is in labour or in the process of abortion.

How much can one rely on investigations in a case of abdominal pain in pregnancy?

Simple investigations can sometimes be very useful in diagnosing the cause of abdominal pain. A microscopic examination of urine may reveal the presence of pus cells and bacteria, suggesting urinary infection. The presence of significant crystals will indicate calculous disease. Culture of the urine with antibiogram is very useful to treat urinary infections.

Microscopic examination of the stool or stool concentrate will help to diagnose amebiasis or worm infestations causing colic. Culture of the stool may yield shigella or salmonella.

Ultrasonography can help to identify most of the obstetric causes of pain as well as some gynecological and surgical causes. It can also detect fibroids or ovarian cysts which are not clinically detected, minimum to moderate free fluid in the peritoneal cavity, stones in the gall bladder, kidney or urinary bladder or gas under the diaphragm.

Radiological investigations are best avoided in pregnancy. They are more harmful in early pregnancy and may not be very useful in late pregnancy. X-rays may be useful only in selected cases, like some cases of calculous urinary disease.

Biochemical investigations and hematological investigations are likely to be helpful to assess the general condition. However, they may not be useful in diagnosing the cause of pain. Even specific tests like serum amylase levels may be raised in pregnancy.

Specific tests like endoscopy or chest skiagram may be done as indicated.

MANAGEMENT

 How does one proceed to manage a patient with the above symptoms?

Treatment will depend on the cause. When medical treatment is prescribed, the guidelines on the use of drugs in pregnancy should be kept in mind. However, the necessary drug should be prescribed if withholding it is likely to worsen the mother's condition. For dyspepsia and heartburn, the pregnant women must be instructed to avoid fatty foods but consume small carbohydrate-rich meals. She should be advised to rest in a propped-up position and avoid lying supine. Symptomatic relief should be given due consideration; the use of antacids and antispasmodics may relieve pain and anxiety. A combination of magnesium trisilicate (500 mg) and aluminium hydroxide (250 mg) is the first line of treatment. Proprietary antacids containing anticholinergic agents may be used when necessary. Cimetidine, ranitidine and other H_2 blockers cross the placental barrier. The safety of long-acting H_2 blockers and omeprazole has not been established in human pregnancy.

A pregnant woman is likely to complain of abdominal pain due to constipation. She must be advised to consume a high fibre diet (vegetables and fruits). Laxatives may be prescribed if constipation is not relieved.

Wherever possible, surgical treatment may be postponed until after the delivery. Routine elective surgical treatment and anesthesia during pregnancy are associated with significant increase in morbidity. However, in acute conditions, one may have to resort to emergency surgical measures. In advanced pregnancy, a cesarean section should not be performed along with surgery for acute conditions in the absence of an obstetric indication. Examples are acute appendicitis, perforation of hollow viscus and intestinal obstruction. There is a significant rise in morbidity of the mother if the two procedures are combined.

Certain conditions like ovarian cyst with pregnancy will require surgical treatment to prevent the occurrence of an acute complication. In such situations, it is ideal to operate in the second trimester when there are likely to be minimum complications. There is a possibility of abortion or preterm labour following such treatment.

Key points

1. Abdominal pain during pregnancy is a common symptom due to uterine enlargement or uterine contractions.
2. Gastroesophageal reflux leads to 'heartburn' in a significant number of pregnant women.
3. Remember that pain could be due to obstetric, gynecologic, surgical and medical disorders.
4. The detection of non-obstetric causes is particularly difficult in the advanced stage of pregnancy.
5. Whenever a laparotomy is performed for an acute abdominal problem near term, concurrent cesarean section should be resorted to only for obstetric indications.

CHAPTER 11

Jaundice in pregnancy

ASHA OUMACHIGUI
APARNA AGRAWAL

Jaundice in pregnancy may result from liver diseases either peculiar to pregnancy or incidental to it. Areas of concern in obstetric practice are the adverse effects on the pregnant woman and her fetus. In India, infective hepatitis is the commonest cause of jaundice; it accounts for 8–10 per cent of all maternal deaths.

Objectives

At the end of this chapter, the reader should be able to

- ❏ Define jaundice.
- ❏ Enumerate the common causes of jaundice during pregnancy.
- ❏ Interpret the information gathered from history and physical examination.
- ❏ Select appropriate investigations and interpret the results.
- ❏ Enumerate the adverse effects of hepatitis on the mother and the fetus.
- ❏ Plan appropriate treatment.
- ❏ Refer effectively cases of jaundice with pregnancy, to tertiary care institutions.

CLINICAL SCENARIO

A 26-year-old primigravida presents with jaundice at 32 weeks of pregnancy.

HISTORY

 What are the aspects one should look at in order to gain a better understanding of the symptoms?

1. Jaundice refers to yellow discolouration of the skin, sclera and mucous membrane due to excessive bilirubin concentration in the body fluids (normal serum bilirubin in pregnancy is 2–17 μmol/l). In this case, the jaundice has appeared in the third trimester and could be due to *acute fatty liver of pregnancy (AFLP), severe pre-eclampsia* charecterised by hemolysis, elevated liver enzymes and low platelets *(HELLP syndrome)* or *viral hepatitis.*

2. Other symptoms are loss of appetite, failure to gain weight or loss of weight, and extreme fatigue.

3. *Fever* is mild and precedes jaundice in viral hepatitis. Fever associated with jaundice may be seen in malaria, leptospirosis, salmonella or disseminated tuberculosis.

4. Right upper quadrant or *epigastric pain* is mild in viral hepatitis. In HELLP syndrome or eclampsia, the pain is severe and is caused by subcapsular hemorrhage in the liver.

5. *Pruritus* is associated with jaundice in the cholestatic phase of viral hepatitis. It is also encountered in intrahepatic cholestasis of pregnancy, biliary obstruction and alcoholic hepatitis.

6. *Urine*—One must enquire about yellowish colour of urine; it turns dark on standing as urobilin is formed.

7. *Stools*—The patient may complain of diarrhea in the prodromal phase of acute viral hepatitis. The stool may be clay-coloured in obstructive type of jaundice.

8. *Drugs*—Toxicity due to drugs like paracetamol and sodium valproate may result in jaundice. Use of tetracyclines is likely to precipitate AFLP.

9. *Family history* of jaundice is obtained in almost half of the women suffering from intrahepatic cholestasis of pregnancy (IHCP). It is due to genetic predisposition and is also due to an increased sensitivity to sex steroids with altered membrane composition of bile ducts and hepatocytes.

10. *Risk factors*—One must enquire about transfusion of blood and blood products, history of any infections, contact with jaundiced patients (especially within the household), sexual contact with an HBV carrier and travel to areas where hepatitis is endemic. Personnel working as paramedical/medical staff handling blood and body fluids are at risk of contracting hepatitis.

EXAMINATION

General examination

The patient is likely to appear very ill in case of hyperemesis gravidarum, HELLP syndrome and acute hepatitis. Dehydration is characteristic of hyperemesis. Pallor due to anemia is noted if jaundice is due to hemolysis.

The presence of hypertension and edema points to pre-eclampsia; these two signs are also associated with AFLP.

Purpuric spots or mucosal bleed, if present, indicate HELLP syndrome, AFLP or fulminant hepatitis. Spider angiomas and palmar erythema may be present in normal pregnant women and are not necessarily indicative of an underlying liver disorder.

Systemic examination

Splenomegaly may be present whenever there is hemolysis, or if the patient is also suffering from malaria or salmonella infection. If the liver is not palpable, the liver dullness should be checked. If it is reduced, the patient may be going into fulminant hepatic failure.

Whenever ascites is present with jaundice, Budd–Chiari syndrome and chronic liver disease should be ruled out.

Obstetric examination

This is performed to assess the period of gestation, fetal status, and to plan the mode of delivery.

DIFFERENTIAL DIAGNOSIS

The following are the most plausible causes of jaundice in the case under discussion.
Viral hepatitis A* to *E—It remains the most common cause of jaundice in pregnancy and accounts for 50–60 per cent of cases in India as the disease is endemic. During epidemics, the incidence of the disease could be much higher.

Since clinical presentations overlap, specific diagnosis is possible only on detection of specific serological markers of acute and chronic infection.

Transmission is from person to person via feco-oral route, transfusion of blood, reused syringes and needles and sexual contact. In acute infection in pregnancy or during delivery, vertical transmission may occur from mother to child.

Pregnant mothers should be screened for HBsAg. Seropositive mothers should be identified and their neonates administered hepatitis B immunoglobulins (HBIg) to prevent neonatal infection.

There is no contraindication to administration of HBIg and a licensed hepatitis B vaccine to pregnant mothers.

It is important to remember that delivery by cesarean section, immediate separation of the baby from the mother and avoidance of breast-feeding do not prevent infection. There is no contraindication to breast-feeding.

Intrahepatic cholestasis of pregnancy—IHCP is second only to viral hepatitis as a cause of jaundice in pregnancy. Generalised pruritus, mild jaundice and intrahepatic cholestasis occur characteristically in the third trimester. Itching becomes increasingly severe and is relieved within 48 hours of delivery.

Liver disorder in pre-eclampsia and eclampsia—Some patients with pre-eclampsia in the third trimester may present principally with hepatic dysfunction and HELLP syndrome.

Subcapsular hemorrhages in the liver are known to occur in pre-eclampsia and eclampsia.

Acute fatty liver of pregnancy—This condition occurs typically in obese women. The predilection is for primigravidae; common independent associations are pre-eclampsia and multiple pregnancy. Maternal and fetal mortality are high.

Drug toxicities—Drugs causing hepatotoxicity include commonly used drugs like paracetamol, isoniazid, rifampicin, tetracyclines, methyl dopa and tricyclic antidepressants. Hepatotoxicity of the fetal liver can occur from metabolites of paracetamol leading to impaired coagulation and intraventricular hemorrhage.

Liver disorder in hyperemesis gravidarum—Excessive vomiting sufficient to require hospitalisation may lead to hepatic dysfunction. The adverse effects of dehydration and starvation are responsible for liver injury. The liver dysfunction responds to control of vomiting and correction of dehydration.

INVESTIGATIONS

Laboratory investigations are absolutely essential and are performed with the aim of determining the cause of jaundice and assessing the severity of liver dysfunction.

Biochemical investigations

Alkaline phosphatase increases during pregnancy whereas lactic dehydrogenase (LDH), aspartate and alanine aminotransferases (AST and ALT) rise during labour. Serum albumin decreases whereas serum lipids increase in pregnancy.

❖ Urine—Bile salts and pigments are present in hepatocellular or cholestatic jaundice. Urobilinogen is raised in hemolytic jaundice.

❖ Blood—Raised serum levels of AST and ALT are seen in hepatic dysfunction, even before the manifestation of jaundice.

Raised levels of AST, ALT and LDH with a reduced platelet count is characteristic of HELLP syndrome.

Serological tests—These are performed to determine the viral markers for the type of hepatitis. HBsAg, anti-HBc (IgM), HBeAg and antibodies to HCV, HDV and HEV are useful. Screening of all pregnant mothers for HBsAg has been advocated so that neonatal immunoprophylaxis can be given to babies of seropositive mothers.

Specific investigations for malaria, salmonella and leptospira infection should be conducted in selected cases.

Imaging techniques

Serial ultrasonography must be performed for suspected liver hematoma, infarction and hepatic rupture. Computerised axial tomography (CAT) scan and magnetic resonance imaging (MRI) may be required. These techniques are also useful in AFLP.

MANAGEMENT

 How does one proceed to manage this patient?

Supportive—The first step in the management of a pregnant woman suffering from jaundice, is to provide *supportive* therapy by combating hypoglycemia and aggravating factors, and monitoring the patient's fluid and dietary intake to ensure that the patient's weight and hydration are maintained.

❖ Strict bed rest advised

❖ Reduced dietary protein intake

❖ Reduced intestinal ammoniagenic substrates

❖ High carbohydrate nutrition (200–300 g of glucose per day)

❖ Administer antipruritic agents. Cholestyramine has been used with good results.

❖ Monitor prothrombin time as it is the most sensitive indicator of the severity of liver dysfunction.

Obstetric management

Obstetric management depends on the condition of the patient. Immediate termination of pregnancy by cesarean section if labour is not imminent, is indicated in AFLP and HELLP syndrome as postpartum recovery is rapid.

Preterm delivery has been reported in half of the patients suffering from jaundice. The risk of postpartum hemorrhage due to coagulation failure is high and every measure should be taken to deal with it. Fresh blood and blood products should be available to support any surgical intervention, and following delivery, to minimise or compensate blood loss. Parenteral administration of vitamin K and folinic acid has been advocated routinely.

The patient should be referred to a higher centre for the following indications:

✤ Altered sensorium
✤ Coagulopathy
✤ Shrinking liver
✤ Non-availability of plasma factors

Key points

1. Viral hepatitis is the commonest cause of jaundice during pregnancy.
2. The detection of viral markers in the serum helps to distinguish viral hepatitis from AFLP and IHCP.
3. Severe pre-eclampsia is frequent and therefore the possibility of HELLP syndrome should be considered.
4. Biochemical and serological tests are essential for accurate diagnosis and logical management.
5. The chances of preterm delivery are high.
6. Coagulation failure precipitates the risk of postpartum hemorrhage.
7. Termination of pregnancy definitely improves maternal outcome in AFLP and HELLP syndrome and intrahepatic cholestasis of pregnancy.
8. Pregnant women should be screened for HBsAg; if positive, the neonate should be given immunoprophylaxis.
9. There are no specific contraindications to administering HBIg and licensed hepatitis B vaccine during pregnancy.
10. Breast-feeding is not contraindicated.

CHAPTER 12

Vaginal bleeding in late pregnancy

P. REDDI RANI

Antepartum hemorrhage (APH) is a complication of pregnancy where the bleeding occurs from or into the genital tract after the 28th week of pregnancy but before the birth of the baby. Along with other causes of obstetric hemorrhage, it contributes to significant maternal and fetal morbidity and mortality.

Objectives

At the end of this chapter, the reader should be able to

- ❑ Define antepartum hemorrhage.
- ❑ Enumerate important causes of APH.
- ❑ Differentiate clinically between placenta previa and abruptio placentae.
- ❑ Select relevant investigations.
- ❑ Enumerate common complications.
- ❑ Plan the management of a case of APH appropriately, institute immediate treatment and refer appropriately.

CLINICAL SCENARIO

A second gravida at 34 weeks of gestation presents with bleeding per vaginum.

HISTORY

What questions should be asked to gain more information regarding the symptoms with which the patient is presenting?

1. *Bleeding per vaginum*—An attempt should be made to find out the amount of bleeding. It is important to ask if the patient had similar episodes earlier. If the answer is yes, the bleeding is said to be recurrent and this is characteristic of placenta previa. In this condition, the placenta is implanted on the lower segment (Fig. 12.1), and covers the os partially or completely. Whenever the lower segment stretches, the placenta comes adrift from its attachment. This process is further enhanced by the downward pressure of the presenting part on the membranes or the placenta (Fig. 12.2). Hemorrhage is inevitable in this condition. The colour of blood in placenta previa is bright red, unlike in accidental hemorrhage where it is dark.

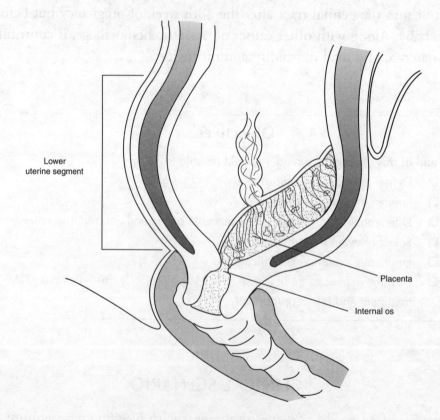

Lower
uterine segment

Placenta

Internal os

Fig. 12.1 Placenta in the lower segment

The initial hemorrhage in placenta previa is small and is called the 'warning hemorrhage' which **must never be ignored. The bleeding is usually painless, causeless and recurrent.**

The other cause for bleeding is an abnormal separation of a normally situated placenta — abruptio placentae also known as **accidental hemorrhage**. Bleeding is retroplacental, not all of it is revealed and by the time the blood trickles down, it is altered and appears dark.

Sometimes the bleeding is due to rupture of a fetal blood vessel which lies below the presenting part; this condition is vasa previa.

2. ***Pain***—Beginning of intermittent colicky *pain* suggests onset of labour. If there is discharge of blood with mucus, it may be 'show'. If the quantity of blood is more, a careful evaluation is warranted.

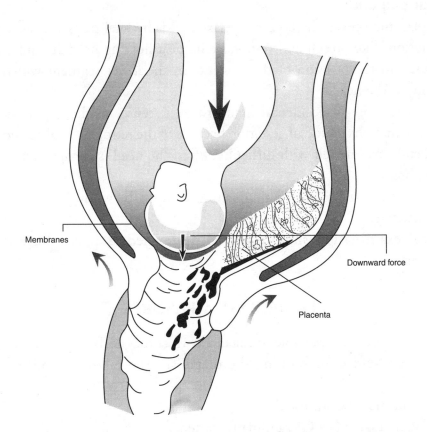

Fig. 12.2 Mechanism of bleeding in placenta previa: shearing mechanism

Continuous severe pain occurs in abruptio placentae. Retroplacental bleeding stretches the uterus to produce pain.

3. Symptoms suggestive of *PIH* are found in 15–30 per cent of women with abruptio placentae.

EXAMINATION

General examination

Pallor, tachycardia and hypotension are directly proportional to the amount of blood loss. In cases of accidental hemorrhage, the above features are out of proportion to the visible blood loss; edema and hypertension could be associated with accidental hemorrhage.

Abdominal palpation

In case of placenta previa, the uterus is relaxed and the fetal parts are easily palpable. Malpresentations like breech and transverse lie or a floating head are quite frequent, and attributed to the position of the placenta in the lower segment which prevents 'stabilisation' of the head.

The uterus in case of accidental hemorrhage is tense, tender, rigid and may be enlarged more than the period of gestation because of the retroplacental accummulation of blood. Fetal parts are felt with difficulty; often the head is engaged and fetal heart sounds are absent.

Table 11.1 summarises the distinguishing features between placenta previa and abruptio placentae.

A vaginal examination should not be performed as it can have disastrous consequences.

IMMEDIATE MEASURES

Clinically, it is not always possible to make a correct diagnosis. However, in a patient with APH even **before** establishing the diagnosis, the following measures should be taken:

❖ The patient must be admitted.

❖ IV line with a large (18 G) cannula is started.

❖ Blood is sent for cross-matching.

Table 12.1

Clinical features	Placenta previa	Abruptio placentae
Nature of bleeding	Painless, causeless and recurrent Bleeding is always revealed	Bleeding may be concealed or revealed painful
Colour of blood	Bright red	Dark red
Deterioration in general condition	Proportionate to amount of blood loss	Out of proportion to visible blood loss in concealed type
Features of PIH	Absent	Present in a third of cases
Abdominal examination		
Height of uterus	Proportionate to gestational period	More than the gestational period due to accumulation of blood
Feel of uterus	Soft and relaxed	May be tense, tender and rigid
Malpresentation	Common. Head may be floating.	Usually vertex, head may be engaged
Fetal heart sounds	Usually present	Absent in concealed type or severe revealed type

❖ Ringer lactate is administered to replenish the circulatory volume, till blood is available.

❖ The patient is sedated.

❖ **Every case of bleeding in late pregnancy is presumed to be placenta previa until otherwise proved.**

After instituting resuscitative measures, the patient should be referred to an institution where facilities for further investigation and management are available.

INVESTIGATIONS

These are done after resuscitative measures:

1. *Ultrasonography* is essential for localisation of placenta. The presence of placenta in the lower segment confirms the diagnosis of placenta previa. It is of minor degree if it just reaches the os and of a major degree if it covers the os partially or completely.

2. If the placenta is normally situated, look for retroplacental clots. The period of gestation and fetal well-being should be assessed in addition to placental localisation.

3. *Other investigations* such as hemogram, bleeding and clotting time, and clot retraction time must be done in all cases of APH. Assessment of plasma fibrinogen and fibrin degradation products are essential. Urinalysis must be done for presence of proteins.

MANAGEMENT OF PLACENTA PREVIA

An expectant line of management is instituted with the objective of continuing the pregnancy till 37 weeks so as to reduce perinatal morbidity and mortality due to prematurity. This line of management should be interrupted if:

❖ Pregnancy reaches 37 weeks.
❖ There is excessive bleeding.
❖ Fetus is dead or malformed.
❖ Labour begins.

The indications for termination of expectant line of management should be strictly adhered to in the interest of both the mother and her fetus.

The mode of termination of pregnancy is cesarean in case of major degree placenta previa. In minor degree placenta previa, **oxytocin drip must be preceded by artificial rupture of membranes in order to prevent further placental separation and hemorrhage.** The management is summarised in the flow chart given in the next page.

How does one proceed to manage a patient with abruptio placentae?

The principle guiding the management of accidental hemorrhage is to institute immediate delivery. To a great extent this measure will prevent DIC and renal failure in the mother. Delivery can be achieved by an ARM and oxytocin drip. Cesarean section is indicated under the following circumstances.

❖ Abruption at term pregnancy with a live fetus
❖ Non-progress of labour for 6–8 hours with ARM and oxytocin on

Remember that both **placenta previa and abruptio placentae predispose to postpartum hemorrhage** (PPH).

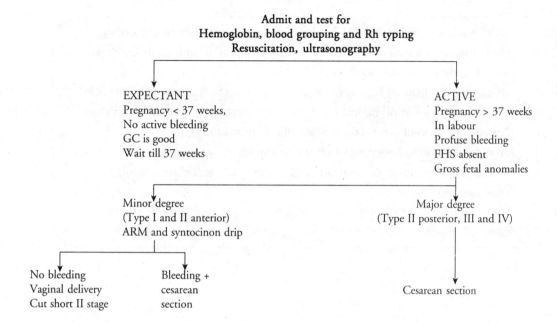

In placenta previa PPH is caused by:
- Imperfect retraction of the lower uterine segment
- Large surface area of placenta with atonic uterus
- Adherent placenta

In abruptio placentae PPH is caused by
- Uterine atonicity
- Coagulation failure
- Couvelaire uterus

Therefore in all cases of APH, one should anticipate PPH. Active management of the third stage is essential to prevent PPH. If it occurs, prompt treatment with IV methergin, oxytocin infusion (10–40 units) and IM 15-methyl $PGF_{2\alpha}$ 250 µg, with simultaneous resuscitation and blood replacement is called for.

Key points

1. In 70 per cent of cases, the cause of antepartum hemorrhage is placenta previa or abruptio placentae.

2. In placenta previa the bleeding is painless, causeless and recurrent. In abruptio placentae, the vaginal bleeding may be revealed or concealed with severe abdominal pain and may be associated with PIH.

3. Pelvic examination should **NOT** be done in cases of antepartum hemorrhage unless placenta previa is excluded by ultrasonographic examination, as it can precipitate dangerous hemorrhage.

4. Expectant management has no place in case of abruptio placentae, whereas in placenta previa it should be instituted when the period of gestation is less than 37 weeks, to prevent perinatal mortality due to prematurity.

5. Rapid delivery is the treatment of choice in abruptio placentae.

6. The two major maternal complications of abruptio placentae are coagulation failure and renal failure.

7. Significant perinatal mortality in APH is due to prematurity and intrauterine death.

CHAPTER 13

Swelling of feet during pregnancy

S. Soundara Raghavan

Swelling of the lower limbs in the absence of hypertension is a common occurrence during pregnancy, particularly after the second trimester. Increased water retention is a normal physiological alteration in pregnancy and is mediated by a fall in plasma osmolarity. In addition, in late pregnancy, increased mechanical obstruction to the venous return from lower limbs (by the enlarging uterus) enhances edema. The reaction of the pregnant woman to swelling of her feet may vary from totally ignoring it to anxiety even when the swelling is mild and probably physiological. While a number of women may experience the so called physiological edema, it is wise to remember that it can be a manifestation of serious conditions like pregnancy-induced hypertension (PIH) and heart disease. The obstetrician rendering antenatal care should be alert enough to detect edema in the early stage and look for an underlying disorder, so that disastrous consequences can be avoided.

Objectives

At the end of this chapter, the reader should be able to

- ❑ Enumerate the causes of swelling of feet during pregnancy.
- ❑ Detect edema of feet.
- ❑ Distinguish physiological edemá from pathological edema.
- ❑ Obtain relevant history from antenatal mothers who present with swelling of feet.
- ❑ Perform necessary clinical examination to identify the cause of swelling of feet.

> ❑ Request appropriate investigations.
> ❑ Institute rational treatment.
> ❑ Counsel mothers with edema; explain and allay apprehension when
>   edema is physiological.

CLINICAL SCENARIO

*A 20-year-old primigravida at 32 weeks of gestation presents with swelling of feet of
one month duration.*

HISTORY

 *What questions should be asked to gain a better understanding of the
case?*

1. It is necessary to obtain *further history* about the swelling of feet. The pregnant
    mother may be asked whether the swelling of feet persists all the time or it appears
    during a particular time of the day. Physiological edema is usually maximum by
    the end of the day. It is relieved by rest. Swelling of feet not relieved by rest or
    found early in the morning, is likely to be pathological.

    One must think of PIH, as the first possibility in a pregnant woman. The incidence
    of PIH is about 8–11 per cent. In congestive cardiac failure, and anemia with
    hypoproteinemia, edema is first seen only in dependant parts. However, in these
    two conditions the presenting symptom is predominantly breathlessness (see
    Chapter 7).

2. *Association of swelling elsewhere in the body*—History may be elicited regarding
    the swelling of feet associated with swelling of other parts of body. Physiological
    edema usually occurs in the dependant parts like feet or the small of the back.
    Presence of edema in non-dependant parts like the face could be due to renal
    disease, in the upper limbs due to mediastinal tumours and in the vulva due to
    pelvic pathology. Presence of edema in non-dependant parts is certainly abnormal.

    An increasing degree of edema involving other parts of the body is an indicator of
    severity of disease like pre-eclampsia or hypoproteinemia associated with malnutrition.

Is it possible to diagnose edema before it manifests clinically?

Careful questioning may reveal that the amount of urine passed is reduced, before the edema manifests clinically. Some women may also state that they feel heavier; others realise that their toe rings or bangles become tighter. If a weight chart is being recorded in the antenatal card, it may be noted that the rate of weight gain exceeds the normal gain of 500 g per week and the weight gain occurs suddenly. At this stage, it is referred to as *occult edema.* It is therefore mandatory to maintain a meticulous weight chart as part of antenatal care. Any increase in weight gain exceeding 500 g per week should be considered as an indicator of occult edema.

 Can edema occur in early pregnancy?

Physiological edema is partly due to reduced venous return from dependant parts and is aggravated by pressure on great vessels by the enlarged uterus. This occurs mostly in the late second or third trimester. Edema occurring in first or early second trimester is considered abnormal and is seen in conditions like multiple pregnancy, hydramnios, and hydatidiform mole, where the uterus is overdistended. The possibility of edema prior to pregnancy due to renal pathology should be kept in mind.

 What are the other relevant points to be obtained during history-taking?

The presence of other symptoms should be enquired into. The woman may have headache and oliguria in case of PIH. Visual disturbances, nausea, vomiting, epigastric pain and irritability are associated with imminent eclampsia; occasionally, eclampsia can occur in the absence of these symptoms.

Symptoms like easy fatiguability, malaise and breathlessness may occur in anemia. History of recurrent UTI may also be present. Significant breathlessness, limitation of activity, palpitations, chest pain, orthopnea and nocturnal dyspnea, cough, and hemoptysis may be found in cardiac disease (see Chapter 8). Parity should be noted; if the patient is a primigravida one must consider pre-eclampsia.

 How does past history help?

If the patient is multiparous, one must enquire about the presence of pre-eclampsia or eclampsia during *previous pregnancy.* Pre-eclampsia can recur in 30 per cent cases.

History of fever with chills and rigors may be obtained in filarial lymphangitis.

History of predisposing causes for anemia, such as dysentery, hemorrhoids, and menorrhagia should be elicited. An enquiry about history suggestive of rheumatic fever, diagnosis of cardiac disease, history of medical and surgical treatment for heart disease will be helpful.

Past history of renal disease like glomerulonephritis or nephrotic syndrome may help to localise the cause to the kidneys. History of jaundice or diagnosis of other liver disorders may indicate edema of hepatic origin.

 What are the relevant points in family history?

An enquiry should be made into the existence of pre-eclampsia among mother and sisters. An association has been noted between the human lymphocyte antigen (HLA) DR4 and proteinuric hypertension.

History of *diabetes mellitus* is relevant as diabetics are more prone to pre-eclampsia.

EXAMINATION

Important points to be noted in the clinical examination

❖ *General*—Edema of the lower limbs is confirmed. It is usually pitting in nature. Presence of unilateral edema of foot or leg occurs due to venous thrombosis or filarial lymphangitis, and the edema is painful. In chronic filariasis, the edema becomes nonpitting.

The degree of pallor is noted. Nutritional anemia is highly prevalent among pregnant women and many of them have associated hypoproteinemia; both of these conditions are responsible for edema.

The blood pressure is recorded carefully. A recording of 140/90 or more on occasions six hours apart, a rise of 30 mm of systolic or 15 mm of diastolic BP above the baseline readings is diagnostic of PIH. This simple examination should always be performed and the results should be interpreted correctly. Blood pressure may be elevated in some renal conditions too. A thorough examination of the cardiovascular system should be performed to rule out an organic heart disease.

❖ *Abdominal examination* should include *checking for ascites and enlarged liver or spleen.* Liver or spleen may be enlarged in cardiac failure or endocarditis. Rarely, the swelling may be caused by a hepatic disorder where there may be ascites or splenomegaly.

❖ *Obstetric examination*—This is performed with the aim of assessing the period of gestation to detect fetal growth restriction. This information is particularly important when one is dealing with PIH as there is a need to assess the fetal wellbeing further. If the fetal wellbeing is compromised or PIH is uncontrolled, termination of pregnancy is indicated and may call for a referral to an institution with a neonatal intensive care unit.

Causes of swelling of feet in pregnancy

Bilateral pitting	Unilateral non-pitting
Physiological	*Tender*
Anemia/hypoproteinemia	Lymphangitis
Pre-eclampsia	Cellulitis
Cardiac disease	Venous thrombosis
Renal disease	*Non-tender*
Hepatic disease	Filarial elephantiasis

INVESTIGATIONS

How should one proceed to investigate a patient with edema feet?

The history and physical examination would be useful in arriving at a provisional diagnosis. If the edema is physiological, there is no need to investigate further. Anemia, heart and hepatic diseases are dealt with elsewhere (see Chapters 8 and 11).

The laboratory investigations are selected essentially to assess the severity and for fetal surveillance.

1. *Hemogram* is useful as in women of low socioeconomic status, anemia and pre-eclampsia coexist. Low platelet count occurs in severe pre-eclampsia.

2. *Urinalysis* should be done. The presence of proteinuria 1 + or more (>300 mg/24 hours) is significant and denotes pre-eclampsia. Proteinuria is also present in renal disease.

3. A *microscopic examination* of the urine points to renal disease if epithelial and granular casts are found. If pus cells are present in significant numbers, a culture must be requested.

4. *Biochemical study* includes estimation of serum uric acid and creatinine. Glucose Tolerance Test is done if there is a family history of diabetes mellitus. A rise in serum uric acid above 6–8 mg per cent is pathological particularly for the fetus.

Serum ALT (SGPT) > 40 units suggests liver dysfunction and is indicative of severe pre-eclampsia.

5. *Ultrasonography and nonstress test are* done for fetal surveillance.

Most of the causes of swelling of feet can be clinically diagnosed. Echocardiography will confirm the diagnosis of cardiac disease and will help to ascertain the severity.

Liver function tests may help to identify liver disease. Ultrasonography of liver and kidneys may be done as required.

MANAGEMENT

 How does one manage a case of pre-eclampsia?

The first measure to be adopted is hospitalisation, irrespective of whether the patient has mild (BP 140/90 mmHg) or severe (160/110) pre-eclampsia.

1. *Rest* in left lateral position, has been found to be beneficial for both the mother and her fetus.

2. *Anti-hypertensives* should be prescribed. The commonly used drugs are alphamethyl dopa at a dose of 250 mg sixth hourly to start with. Calcium channel blockers like nifedipine 5 mg is given sublingually in severe pre-eclampsia. ACE inhibitors are contraindicated; so are diuretics as both these are *harmful* to the fetus.

3. *Termination* of pregnancy is the most specific *treatment* for pre-eclampsia. In the interest of both the mother and the fetus, pregnancy should be terminated definitely by 37 weeks. Pregnancy should be terminated earlier if the severity of pre-eclampsia cannot be controlled, irrespective of the period of gestation.

Key points

1. Edema feet occurs in about 30 per cent of pregnant women.
2. It is caused by excessive water retention and pressure on the pelvic veins by the enlarged uterus. Physiological edema disappears after rest.
3. Pathological edema is associated with PIH. It is also seen in severe anemia with hypoproteinemia and congestive cardiac failure.
4. Occult edema is detected whenever there is a sudden weight gain of more than 500 g/week.
5. Blood pressure must be checked at every visit in all pregnant women especially in those with edema.

---

6. If a BP of 140/90 or a rise in systolic BP by 30 mm Hg and diastolic BP by 15 mm Hg is recorded, the patient must be hospitalised and closely monitored.
7. Alphamethyldopa and calcium channel blockers are employed for control of BP.
8. Pregnancy must be terminated by 37 weeks or earlier if indicated.

CHAPTER 14

Hypertension in pregnancy

S. HABEEBULLAH

Hypertensive disorders of pregnancy contribute significantly to maternal morbidity and mortality besides accounting for high perinatal morbidity and mortality. About 7–8% of pregnancies are complicated by hypertension. Maternal mortality due to obstetric hemorrhage has reduced to some extent, but that due to hypertensive disorders has been on the rise. Hypertension is an important cause of intrauterine growth restriction (IUGR), intrauterine death (IUD) and increased obstetric interventions. Uncontrolled hypertension, pre-eclampsia in particular can result in a convulsive disorder that is eclampsia. The disease affects the liver, kidneys and the brain. Though hypertension may not be entirely preventable, the complications can be prevented through early diagnosis and appropriate interventions.

Objectives

At the end of this chapter, the reader should be able to
- ❑ Define hypertension in pregnancy.
- ❑ Classify hypertensive disorders in pregnancy.
- ❑ Obtain relevant history towards proper management.
- ❑ Identify features of severe pre-eclampsia.
- ❑ List maternal and fetal complications
- ❑ Outline the relevant investigations to assess the maternal and fetal condition.
- ❑ Institute emergency management for severe pre-eclampsia.
- ❑ Explain the prognosis to the mothers and counsel them for follow up.

CLINICAL SCENARIO

A 20-year-old primigravida at 34 weeks' pregnancy presents with BP 160/120 mm Hg.

It is essential to know what constitutes hypertension in pregnancy.

Definition of hypertension in pregnancy: A systolic blood pressure (SBP) of 140 mm Hg or more and diastolic BP (DBP) of 90 mm Hg or more recorded at least on two occasions 6 hours apart is considered as hypertension. Mean arterial pressure (MAP) $\geq$ 105 mm Hg or increase in MAP by 20 mmHg is also diagnostic. MAP is calculated using the formula

[SBP + (DBP x 2)] ÷ 3

Hypertension is considered severe if it is $\geq$160/110 mm Hg

Classification: The commonly followed classification of hypertension is:

1. Pregnancy induced hypertension (PIH): Hypertension is detected in a pregnant woman who was normotensive before pregnancy.
   a) Pre-eclampsia (with proteinuria > 300 mg in 24 h urine)
   b) Eclampsia (with convulsions)
2. Chronic or preexisting hypertension (existing before pregnancy)
3. Pre-eclampsia/eclampsia superimposed on chronic hypertension
4. Transient hypertension—developing near term or early puerperium with rapid resolution
5. Unclassified

Sometimes the term *gestational hypertension* is used for those who develop hypertension (without proteinuria) during pregnancy; their blood pressure returns to normal after delivery.

The patient in question is suffering from severe hypertension.

 What questions should one ask the above patient?

The hypertensive pregnant woman may or may not be symptomatic. In many cases hypertension may be detected during routine antenatal check up. She must be asked whether the hypertension was present before pregnancy or whether it was present in the previous pregnancy. Primigravida and obese women are at an increased risk of pre-eclampsia. History of excess weight gain and/or pathological edema may be present. Symptoms of severe hypertension like headache and oliguria should be noted. Hypertension along with persistent headache usually frontal, blurring of vision and epigastric pain suggest imminent eclampsia.

What is the relevance of time of onset of hypertension in pregnancy?

Pregnancy induced hypertension (PIH) is usually a disease of late third trimester. If it is detected before 32 weeks of pregnancy, it is termed early onset PIH, and carries a poorer prognosis. If it is detected before 20 weeks especially in early pregnancy, it is likely to be chronic hypertension. The onset of pre-eclampsia may be earlier in vesicular mole, multiple pregnancy, renal disease and antiphospholipid antibody syndrome.

 Is past medical history important?

It is necessary to check if the patient has diabetes mellitus, hypertension, renal disease, autoimmune diseases like systemic lupus erythematosus (SLE) for which she may be taking treatment.

 What are the points to be noted in the family history?

One must enquire about history of PIH in the mother or sisters; family history of hypertension, renal disease, diabetes mellitus and connective tissue disorders, SLE and antiphospholipid syndrome are relevant.

 What should one look for in general examination?

The most important finding is hypertension. The BP should be checked at every antenatal visit with a view to diagnose hypertension early.

✤ Weight gain should be monitored; a gain of over 500 grams per week must put one on guard.

✤ In most cases PIH develops after 32 weeks of gestation.

✤ Though pedal edema is not diagnostic of pre-eclampsia, pathological edema in non-dependent areas like face, fingers, abdominal wall and vulva should be looked for.

 While performing obstetric examination, what points should one note?

✤ Height of the uterine fudus may be less than that indicated for period of gestation (POG) if hypertension is of significant duration as it may affect fetal growth, especially if PIH is severe. Another reason for this is the decrease in the volume of amniotic fluid.

✤ One should look for multiple pregnancy or molar pregnancy by palpation.

✤ In some cases of severe PIH, ascites may be present.

What investigations should one request for the patient?

Laboratory investigations form an essential part of assessment of pre-eclampsia. They help to identify the severity of the disease. They need to be repeated to assess amelioration or deterioration of the disease. Since pre-eclampsia is characterised by a generalised vasospasm, multiple organs are affected and the investigations should be directed to evaluate the function of all the systems.

❖ Ophthalmoscopic (fundoscopy) examination could detect the severity of vasospasm. In severe cases retinal hemorrhages, retinal detachment and papilledema are seen. These changes are usually reversed after delivery.

❖ Renal: Check 24-hour urinary output, urine for protein, pus cells, casts, culture and sensitivity, blood urea, serum creatinine and uric acid. A 24-hour urinary output less than 500 ml, serum creatinine level more than 1.2 mg/dl and proteinuria over 5 g/24 h indicate severe PIH. Serum uric acid more than 6.5 mg/dl is associated with adverse perinatal outcome.

❖ Liver: SGOT, SGPT, lactic dehydrogenase (LDH) to assess hepatic involvement

❖ Hematological: Hemoglobin and hematocrit, clotting time, platelet count, plasma fibrinogen, fibrinogen degradation products (FDP), peripheral smear for evidence of hemolysis; prothrombin time and activated partial thromboplastin time

Depending on the response to treatment, these investigations may be repeated at least weekly.

❖ Tests for fetal well-being include:
  ▶ Daily Fetal Movement Count (DFMC)
  ▶ Non-stress test (NST) twice weekly
  ▶ Ultrasonography for amount of liquor and other biophysical parameters at least weekly; for assessment of fetal growth every 2 weeks

It is very important to be alert to the possible occurrence of HELLP syndrome as it is associated with a very poor prognosis for the mother and the unborn child.

 What is HELLP syndrome?

Hemolysis, elevated liver enzymes and low platelet count constitute HELLP syndrome. This occurs in 3–5 per cent of cases of severe pre-eclampsia and eclampsia and is associated with high maternal and perinatal mortality. This condition results in mild elevation of serum bilirubin, LDH levels (>600 IU/L) and AST and ALT levels. The platelet count drops to <100,000/cu mm.

What are the other complications one should anticipate?

Other major maternal complications of pre-eclampsia include eclampsia, pulmonary edema, cardiac failure, cerebral hemorrhage, abruptio placentae and coagulation failure due to disseminated intravascular coagulation (DIC) and acute renal failure.

 What are the perinatal complications?

Intrauterine growth restriction, IUD, preterm delivery and its associated complications are common. These complications are exaggerated in chronic hypertension with superimposed pre-eclampsia. Placental abruption also contributes to poor perinatal outcome.

 How does one manage the above patient?

It is best to admit the patient for bed rest and to assess the severity of PIH. Since in PIH the hypertension is labile, a single BP reading in the OPD may not be reliable and representative. BP should be measured every six hours. Though the complications usually follow severe pre-eclampsia, sometimes a patient with mild disease may deteriorate quickly and develop eclampsia or other serious complications like abruption. In rare cases, when the PIH is mild, the patient is willing and likely to attend OPD twice weekly, preferably to a day care unit, ambulatory treatment may be considered. The treatment is along the following lines:

❖ **Bed rest** in lateral position improves uteroplacental perfusion.

❖ **Diet** should include adequate proteins; normal intake of salt is permitted.

❖ **Diuretics** should be avoided as they worsen hemoconcentration and may cause neonatal thrombocytopenia. They are indicated if the patient develops pulmonary edema.

❖ **Antihypertensives** have a role in severe hypertension when the BP is greater than or equal to 160/110 mm Hg. Generally, when the diastolic BP is ≥ 100 mm Hg and pregnancy needs to be prolonged in order to avoid the risks of prematurity, antihypertensives are used. They are likely to reduce maternal complications like cerebrovascular accidents. It should be remembered that bringing down the pressure to normal levels is likely to decrease placental perfusion resulting in fetal death. It is better to keep DBP at 85–90 mm Hg. Long-term studies show that alpha methyldopa is safe in a dose of 250 mg 6 hourly upto 2 g/day. If BP is not under control, nifedipine 10 mg eight hourly upto 120 mg daily can be added.

Alternatively, labetalol 200 mg TID may be given upto a maximum dose of 2400 mg/ day. ACE inhibitors (captopril) are contraindicated in pregnancy, as their use has been associated with IUGR, renal agenesis, hypocalvaria, oligohydramnios and intrauterine death of fetus.

If diastolic BP is $\geq$ 110 mmHg, sublingual nifedipine 5 mg doses may be used to prevent complications like cerebrovascular accident. Labetalol 50 mg IV statum followed by 50 mg/h up to maximum 300 mg may be used. Hydralazine 5–10 mg IV every 30 minutes can also be used if available.

 ### *What is the role of termination of pregnancy in PIH?*

Delivery is the ultimate cure for PIH. In mild PIH pregnancy can be continued till 38 weeks. However, in severe PIH expectant management may be instituted with a view to continuing the pregnancy to 37–38 weeks. However, if in spite of medical treatment, the disease progresses or complications develop the pregnancy will have to be terminated irrespective of the POG.

Unless other obstetric indications warrant cesarean section, vaginal delivery following induction of labour is preferred. During labour in severe pre-eclampsia, prophylactic magnesium sulphate may be administered along with antihypertensives to prevent eclampsia.

Cervical ripening if needed using prostaglandin E_2 gel followed by artificial rupture of membranes for induction of labour is the usual practice. Augmentation of labour using oxytocin drip may also be undertaken if necessary. The fetus should be closely monitored preferably by electronic fetal monitoring. The second stage of labour is curtailed by instrumental delivery. Epidural anesthesia may be employed for cesarean section unless the platelet counts are low. After delivery close monitoring of BP and urinary output for at least 24 hours is absolutely essential. The antihypertensive dose may be reduced or even stopped depending on the BP.

In early onset PIH if the pregnancy is more than 28 weeks and the patient responds to conservative management, pregnancy can be continued. However if the pregnancy is less than 27 weeks, in view of high maternal morbidity and mortality and poor perinatal outcome, it is better to terminate the pregnancy.

Treatment of HELLP syndrome includes delivery by induction of labour after starting corticosteroids, which need to be continued for 3–4 days after delivery.

What is the long-term prognosis?

❖ The hypertension in PIH should resolve after delivery, latest within 12 weeks postpartum. If it persists, it should be labelled as **chronic hypertension**.

❖ There is an increased risk of pre-eclampsia in a subsequent pregnancy, more so if the onset in the index pregnancy is before 30 weeks.

❖ The long-term risk of developing chronic hypertension is more in those who develop recurrent PIH. Therefore, multiparas with PIH are at a greater risk of chronic hypertension than primigravidas with PIH. The patients should be counselled accordingly and the need for follow up emphasised.

 Is pre-eclampsia preventable?

Since the cause of PIH is largely unknown, attempts to prevent the condition have not been very successful. A number of pharmacological methods have been tried. Calcium supplementation 2 g/day especially in populations with dietary deficiencies was shown to be of some benefit.

Low dose aspirin in doses of 40–80 mg/day has been extensively studied. Collaborative Low dose Aspirin in Pregnancy (CLASP) study however showed no benefit in low-risk group. It might be useful in high-risk patients and those who had pre-eclampsia/eclampsia or those who had early onset PIH in the previous pregnancy.

 Can occurrence of pre-eclampsia be predicted?

Since PIH is not completely preventable, it is prudent to diagnose it early so that the complications are reduced to a great extent. Some of the commonly performed tests are:

Roll-over test: It is performed at about 28 weeks of pregnancy. First the BP is checked in left lateral position. Then the woman is turned supine and if the rise in diastolic BP is >20 mm Hg the test is positive.

Isometric handgrip exercise test: Resting BP in left lateral position is taken. Then she is asked to press maximally an inflated BP cuff for 30 seconds. Then she compresses the BP cuff at 50 per cent of the maximum contraction for three minutes. An increase in diastolic BP of 20 mm Hg or more is considered positive pressor response.

Calcium/creatinine ratio: In pre-eclampsia, urinary excretion of calcium is reduced. A calcium/creatinine ratio < 0.04 is considered significant.

Doppler ultrasound: Presence of diastolic notch in the uterine artery doppler in the second trimester of pregnancy predicts development of PIH.

Most of the predictive tests have good negative predictive value; likelihood of developing PIH is low if the test is negative.

 ### How does chronic hypertension affect pregnancy?

Chronic hypertension existing before pregnancy or diagnosed in early pregnancy (before 20 weeks) occurs in about 2% of pregnancies. In about 20–30% of these, there is a risk of superimposed pre-eclampsia. The risk of abruptio placentae and IUGR is also increased. Investigations should be directed to rule out the causes of hypertension. Management is along similar lines. If the patient is already on drugs like ACE inhibitors or atenolol, they should be stopped and replaced by alpha methyldopa and nifedipine. In mild cases, pregnancy might be continued to 37–38 weeks of gestation. Severe cases and those with superimposed pre-eclampsia need meticulous care in the hospital.

Key points

1. BP ≥ 140/90 mm Hg, recorded six hours apart is considered hypertension during pregnancy and ≥ 160/110 mm Hg is severe hypertension.
2. In pre-eclampsia along with hypertension, there is significant proteinuria (> 300 mg/24 h).
3. The onset of PIH is usually after 20 weeks.
4. The pathophysiology includes generalised vasospasm.
5. Hospitalisation and thorough evaluation by relevant investigations of all the organs likely to be affected is essential.
6. Antihypertensives have a role when diastolic BP is ≥ 100 mm Hg during expectant management.
7. HELLP syndrome carries high maternal and perinatal mortality.
8. In mild cases of hypertension, pregnancy must be terminated at 37–38 weeks; in severe cases, when BP cannot be controlled, pregnancy must be terminated irrespective of the POG. Prophylactic magnesium sulphate should be used during labour.
9. The second stage of labour should be cut short by instrumental delivery.
10. Cesarean section is resorted to if there is an obstetric indication
11. Maternal and fetal outcome are adversely affected in PIH, especially in case of severe pre-eclampsia and its complications.
12. Every effort must be made to detect PIH at an early stage.
13. Pharmacological agents with proven benefits must be used in pregnant women at the risk of developing PIH.

CHAPTER 15

Convulsions during pregnancy

S. HABEEBULLAH

Convulsions during pregnancy are alarming and can be a life-threatening emergency. In India, the most common cause of convulsions in pregnancy is eclampsia, which is also one of the three important causes of maternal mortality. Death due to eclampsia can be prevented by prompt diagnosis and management. Eclampsia itself is preventable if pre-eclampsia is diagnosed early and treated. One must also remember that a pregnant woman could suffer from convulsions due to other causes.

Objectives

At the end of this chapter, the reader should be able to

❑ Enumerate the causes of convulsions in pregnancy.
❑ Institute immediate treatment.
❑ Elicit appropriate history and perform relevant physical examination.
❑ List appropriate investigations.
❑ Outline further management of the case.
❑ List the complications of eclampsia.
❑ Appreciate that eclampsia is preventable.

CLINICAL SCENARIO

An 18-year-old primigravida, presents at 36 weeks of gestation with convulsions.

MANAGEMENT

 How does one proceed to manage this patient?

If a patient with convulsions is encountered in a peripheral area, immediate general measures should be taken to clear the airway, prevent injury and control convulsions. The patient should be referred to a higher institution with details of treatment given clearly in the referral letter.

Causes of convulsions in pregnancy

Eclampsia (the most common cause)

Epilepsy

Cerebrovascular accidents

Trauma (head injury)

Poisoning (strychnine, CNS stimulants)

Metabolic disorders (uremia, electrolyte imbalance, hepatic/renal failure, hypoglycemia)

Drug abuse

Infections (meningitis, encephalitis, cerebral malaria in endemic areas)

Functional

Brain tumours in rare cases

Control of convulsions

All pregnant women with convulsions must be considered eclamptic *until proved otherwise*. Immediate treatment consists of general measures and control of convulsions.

General measures—These include nursing the patient, preferably on a railed cot, with head turned to one side on a flat surface. Airway should be cleared by suction; oral airway or mouth gag is used to prevent the tongue from rolling back and to prevent injuries to the tongue. Oxygen is administered and IV line is secured.

Medication—Simultaneously, steps should be taken to control convulsions. Several drugs like diazepam, and phenytoin have been used, but the drug of choice is magnesium sulphate administered parenterally according to Pritchard's regimen as shown below.

Loading dose of 4 g of $MgSO_4$ (as 20 ml of 20 per cent solution) given IV slowly over five minutes

Additional injection of 2 g of $MgSO_4$ (as 10 ml of 20 per cent solution) if convulsions do not cease, and

Inj of 10 g of MgSO$_4$ (as 10 ml of 50 per cent solution – 5 g into each buttock)

Maintenance dose

Inj of 5 g of MgSO$_4$ (as 10 ml of 50 per cent solution) IM every four hours on alternate buttocks

Before each dose of MgSO$_4$, it should be *ensured* that:

a) patient's breathing is normal, with a respiratory rate of >14/min.

b) knee jerks are present.

c) urine output in the previous four hours is >100 ml.

Magnesium sulphate should be continued for at least 24 hours after the last convulsion or delivery, whichever is later. **During therapy, the patient must be monitored very carefully with regard to respiration, knee jerks and urine output.**

❖ If magnesium sulphate is not available, diazepam may be used. Initially, 10 mg is given IV as bolus, followed by 40 mg in 500 ml of dextrose as a drip titrated at 20–30 drops/min, according to the frequency of convulsions. The use of lytic cocktail regimen is no longer advocated because of the side effects on the mother and the fetus.

❖ Alternatively one may use phenytoin with a loading dose of 15 mg/kg administered intravenously at the rate of 25 mg/min, followed by 300 mg IV, 12 hours later. Maintenance dose is 100 mg IM 4 hourly. The patient should be under cardiac monitoring.

Once the above measures have been taken, a detailed history should be gathered from the patient's attendants.

HISTORY

 What questions must be asked to gain a better understanding of the case?

The information obtained is useful not only for assessing the prognosis in eclampsia, but also for diagnosis, in case the convulsions are not due to eclampsia.

The number and frequency of convulsions, their duration, and the time of the last convulsion should be noted. A description of the convulsion — how it started, progressed and ended and whether it is localised or generalised should be obtained. A history of vomiting, headache, visual disturbance and epigastric pain usually precedes an eclamptic convulsion. Tonic-clonic convulsions of eclampsia are followed by unconsiousness of varying duration. History of hypertension and oliguria is usually present in eclampsia.

One must enquire if the patient has had convulsions since childhood. If the answer is in the affirmative, epilepsy or status epilepticus could be a possible cause.

Fever precedes convulsions in infections like meningitis, encephalitis or cerebral malaria. Information related to metabolic disorders like uremia, electrolyte imbalance, hypoglycemia or hepatic failure, must be obtained. One must remember the possibility of head injury, cerebrovascular accidents, and brain tumours, and an attempt must be made to obtain relevant information. In cerebrovascular accidents, a history of altered sensorium may precede convulsions.

A note must be made regarding the *drugs that the patient may have taken or have been administered for control of convulsions.*

PHYSICAL EXAMINATION

A thorough examination, directed particularly at the nervous system, should be performed. Characteristically, hypertension is detected in eclampsia, and hyperreflexia is elicited by brisk knee jerks. Sometimes, the blood pressure may be normal or marginally high. The pupils should be noted for size and pupillary reflex. There may be injury to the tongue. Localising neurological signs may be present in intracranial hemorrhage. Evidence of head injury and meningitis should be noted. Chest examination should be performed to rule out aspiration pneumonia and pulmonary edema. One should look for evidence of DIC. The fundus should be examined through the ophthalmoscope to look for hemorrhages, exudates and retinal detachment.

INVESTIGATIONS

These should include :
1. Complete blood count, platelet count, clotting time (CT), fibrinogen, and fibrin degradation products (FDP)
2. Serum electrolytes, blood sugar, liver function tests (LFT), renal function tests (RFT) including serum uric acid
3. Urinalysis—proteins, casts, culture and sensitivity

4   x-ray chest, arterial blood gas analysis if pulmonary edema or aspiration pneumonia is suspected

5.   CT scan if head injury, cerebrovascular accidents or intracranial lesion is suspected

CONTROL OF HYPERTENSION

For control of hypertension, sublingual nifedepine 5 mg or hydralazine 5 mg IV may be used. These may be repeated after 20–30 minutes if adequate response is not seen.

FURTHER MANAGEMENT OF ECLAMPSIA

❖ Blood should be obtained for investigations (mentioned earlier) and crossmatching.

❖ The patient should be catheterised for monitoring urine output, and urinalysis is performed.

❖ Ophthalmic funduscopy should be done if not done already.

❖ Patient should be kept nil orally and IV fluids should be given for maintenance. Other causes of convulsions like epilepsy, metabolic disorders, infection and trauma have to be managed by specific measures in consultation with the specialists in the respective fields.

Obstetric management

One must assess the period of gestation, the condition of the fetus and whether the patient is in labour. An ultrasound examination is helpful to assess the fetal condition. For obstetric indication such as fetal distress or CPD, cesarean section should be performed. When vaginal delivery is contemplated, if the cervix is favourable, low rupture of membranes followed by oxytocin augmentation should be performed. If the cervix is not favourable and there is no other compromising factor, cervical ripening with PGE_2 gel followed after six hours by induction of labour with rupture of membranes and oxytocin may be undertaken. The second stage has to be cut short by low or outlet forceps. If the fetus is not viable, injection $PGF_{2\alpha}$ (250 μg IM every three hours) may be given. Alternatively, extraamniotic ethacridine lactate or $PGF_{2\alpha}$ instillation followed by oxytocin infusion may be done. Prophylactic methergin should be avoided. Close monitoring of the patient is essential as postpartum collapse can occur.

PREVENTION OF ECLAMPSIA

Eclampsia can be prevented in a patient with PIH by admitting the patient, and by closely monitoring the BP and reflexes. If hyperreflexia or other symptoms and signs of imminent eclampsia are present, the patient should be promptly treated with magnesium sulphate (as detailed earlier). Pregnancy should be terminated in all patients with PIH if the fetus is mature or salvageable. In other patients, rest and antihypertensive management should be tried with a view to achieve fetal maturity without endangering the mother's life.

In peripheral centres, patients who develop PIH should be diagnosed early by recognising abnormal weight gain of more than 500 g/week, or by rise in blood pressure to 140/90 or more. These patients may be referred promptly to a tertiary care institution.

COMPLICATIONS

During the attack of convulsions, there may be injuries to the patient including tongue bite. The patient may aspirate gastric contents or the tongue may fall backwards blocking the airway. There may be hyperpyrexia in a patient with convulsions. Cerebrovascular accidents like cerebral hemorrhage can occur if the hypertension is not controlled.

The patient with eclampsia may develop abruptio placentae, which can further worsen her condition. Renal failure, disseminated intravascular coagulation (DIC) and postpartum psychosis are some of the other complications of eclampsia.

FOLLOW UP

Hypertension may persist even after delivery. In subsequent pregnancy, there is at least 25 per cent chance of recurrence of PIH. Therefore, these patients should be considered for treatment with low dose aspirin or calcium supplementation starting from 15–16 weeks in the next pregnancy.

Key points

1. Eclampsia is the commonest cause of convulsions in pregnancy.
2. Other causes may be epilepsy, cerebrovascular accidents, meningitis, encephalitis or cerebral malaria.
3. Eclampsia can be prevented by prompt treatment of PIH.
4. Magnesium sulphate is the drug of choice for controlling convulsions.
5. In most cases, the pregnancy has to be terminated.

CHAPTER 16

Watery discharge per vaginum during pregnancy

ASHA OUMACHIGUI

Vaginal discharge, white or watery, from late second trimester of pregnancy onwards is a fairly common problem for which a pregnant mother may seek advice. Most often, the underlying cause is premature rupture of membranes (PROM), that is, rupture of membranes before the onset of labour. The symptom also could be a manifestation of associated conditions like vaginitis or stress urinary incontinence. A firm diagnosis of rupture of membranes is not always easy to make unless amniotic fluid is seen escaping from the cervical canal. The available tests should be used to confirm PROM so that a logical decision is made regarding further management, to strike a balance between fetal prematurity and chorioamnionitis.

Objectives

At the end of this chapter, the reader should be able to

- ❑ Enumerate causes of vaginal discharge during pregnancy.
- ❑ Define PROM.
- ❑ Enlist the risks of PROM.
- ❑ Take a relevant history.
- ❑ Perform clinical examination.
- ❑ Select tests to confirm or rule out the diagnosis of PROM.
- ❑ Select appropriate investigations to institute rational management.
- ❑ Appreciate the principles underlying the management of PROM.
- ❑ Outline the plan of management of PROM.

CLINICAL SCENARIO

A third gravida, 25 years of age presents with history of 8 months of pregnancy and watery discharge.

HISTORY

 ### What questions should be asked in order to gain a better understanding of the case?

One must enquire about the *mode of onset of discharge.* If it was sudden, the cause is likely to be PROM, particularly rupture of forewaters. The discharge is watery.

It is important to find out if there is history of abdominal pain which could point either to the onset of labour or to placental abruption. One must also find out the possibility of cord prolapse. **These are important complications of PROM in which the fetus is in jeopardy.**

1. The vaginal discharge may have started insidiously perhaps a few days *previously.* In such cases, the possibility of high rupture of membranes with a slow leak of amniotic fluid should be kept in mind.

2. Whenever the duration of the symptoms is long, with gradual onset, one must remember to ask the patient if the discharge is related to an increase in intraabdominal pressure such as coughing or sneezing. Stress urinary incontinence is known to occur among some pregnant women.

3. Infections like trichomonal vaginitis could be responsible for vaginal discharge. Here, the nature of discharge is characteristically thin, greenish in colour and associated with itching.

4. One must ask the patient if she has been having *fever.* Its presence denotes infection so frequently associated with prolonged PROM. In some cases, the patient may also complain of malodorous discharge per vaginum.

5. The date of her last menstrual period must be noted correctly. This will help to assess the period of gestation, which is of paramount importance in the management of PROM, particularly if it is preterm.

6. Regarding the present pregnancy, one should enquire about antenatal care with reference to period of amenorrhea at which pregnancy was confirmed or assessed; detection of hydramnios or multiple pregnancy, all of which predispose to PROM.

7. History of PROM or preterm labour in the previous pregnancy would be relevant. Recurrent PROM has been recorded. Evidence of pelvic infection, particularly due to Neisseria gonorrhea or chlamydia if any, points to PROM.

PHYSICAL EXAMINATION

1. While examining the patient, her general condition should be assessed. She may appear uncomfortable if copious discharge is wetting her clothes. Fever and tachycardia may be present if the PROM is of long duration. She may appear toxic in case of severe chorioamnionitis.
2. Abdominal palpation may reveal the fundal height to be less than the period of gestation in a singleton pregnancy, if a good quantity of liquor has already drained. This finding may not be appreciated in multiple pregnancy. The uterus could be tender if chorioamnionitis has set in.
3. A vaginal speculum examination is useful in viewing escape of amniotic fluid through the cervical canal. It also helps to identify local infections. If infection is present, it would be pertinent to collect the discharge and subject it to a microscopic examination for trichomonas vaginalis or candida albicans.
4. Ammoniacal odour may be observed if the discharge is urine due to incontinence.
5. If there is a suggestion of chorioamnionitis, specimens from the cervix and the vagina must be collected for culture.

At this juncture, intervention is instituted. *Vaginal infection* must be treated with specific drugs, for example, metronidazole for trichomonal vaginitis. Appropriate antibiotic therapy should be started after taking cervical and vaginal swab for culture.

If the diagnosis is doubtful, PROM is confirmed by using two simple tests.

1. A smear is made with the discharge on a slide and it is allowed to dry. The ferning pattern is seen if the fluid is amniotic fluid mixed with cervical mucus.
2. Nitrazine test—A test paper impregnated with nitrazine is touched with a drop of the fluid on cotton swab. The change in colour is compared with a standard colour chart to assess the pH of the fluid. A pH above 6.5 is consistent with amniotic fluid due to ruptured membranes.

Once the diagnosis of PROM is confirmed either clinically or by one of the tests mentioned above, further management is planned. The issues that need to be resolved are as follows:

Under what circumstances should the pregnancy be terminated?

1. If the patient is already in the active phase of labour as characterised by complete effacement of the cervix or cervical dilatation of 4 cm or more.
2. In the presence of clinical chorioamnionitis, the pregnancy is terminated irrespective of the period of gestation. Labour should be induced. Cesarean section is performed only for other obstetric indications.
3. In case of fetal malformations not compatible with life
4. Fetal distress
5. Complications like abruptio placentae and cord prolapse

 ### Is there any need to terminate pregnancy immediately if PROM has occurred after 36 weeks?

No. It is well established that the majority of the patients with a favourable cervix go into labour within six hours. Patients with an unfavourable cervix would go into labour within 24 hours. Recent studies have shown that waiting upto 24 hours does not increase the risk of chorioamnionitis or neonatal sepsis. It is important to bear in mind that induction of labour in patients with an unfavourable cervix leads to an increased risk of failed induction and cesarean section. Vaginal examinations should be minimised and performed with aseptic precautions in order to reduce the risk of chorioamnionitis.

 ### What does one do if the membranes rupture before 36 weeks?

1. Immediate delivery is associated with an increased risk of hyaline membrane disease (HMD). However, if the *expectant line of management* is chosen in order to prolong gestation, the chances of the patient developing chorioamnionitis are considerable.
2. The patient needs to be *investigated*. The purpose of performing laboratory investigations is:
   a. To monitor for chorioamnionitis. As mentioned earlier, a total leukocyte count, erythrocyte sedimentation rate and culture of vaginal swab must be carried out every 48 hours.
   b. C-reactive protein (CRP) or an acute phase reactant has been found to be useful as a screening test for subclinical infection. The levels rise 2–3 days before the development of signs of infection.
   c. **Amniotic fluid analysis**—A Gram stain is easy to perform and gives an idea about the nature of organisms. Antibiotics may be started while waiting for

culture and sensitivity reports. A total leukocyte count of >100 cells per microlitre predicts intraamniotic infection.

d.   To assess the fetal condition, a fetal biophysical profile is done. Ultrasonography is not used for diagnosis of PROM.

There is a positive correlation of intraamniotic infection and neonatal sepsis with nonreactive nonstress test (NST) and no fetal breathing movements, or breathing movements lasting for less than 30 seconds, provided the biophysical profile is performed every 24 hours.

PROM between 32 and 36 weeks

1. Labour should be induced, if (a) the period of gestation is beyond 34 weeks and (b) neonatal intensive care unit is available.
2. Expectant management and antibiotics are called for if the cervix is unripe, lung maturity is doubtful and no subclinical infection is seen.

PROM between 28 and 32 weeks

1. Maternal administration of corticosteroids protects the newborn against hyaline membrane disease (HMD), necrotising enterocolitis and intraventricular hemorrhage. The recommended schedule is: four doses of Inj. Dexamethasone 6 mg IM every 12 hours. Alternatively two doses of Inj. Betamethasone 12 mg may be administered at an interval of 12 hours.
2. Maternal administration of phenobarbitone and vitamin K reduce the risk of intraventricular hemorrhage in the newborn.
3. Maternal pulse, temperature and vaginal discharge are monitored for any evidence of infection; if present, termination of pregnancy is warranted.

PROM before 28 weeks

This group of patients has a poor perinatal outcome. However, expectant line of management can be adopted with maternal administration of antibiotics, corticosteroids, phenobarbitone and vitamin K.

Key points

1.   Premature rupture of membranes (PROM) is the commonest cause of watery discharge in pregnancy.
2.   After 36 weeks, the majority of the patients will be in labour within 24 hours.

3. Visualisation of flow of amniotic fluid through cervical os confirms the diagnosis of PROM. In case of doubt the 'fern test' is useful.

4. Ultrasonography is useful to the extent that normal amniotic fluid rules out PROM.

5. The diagnosis of chorioamnionitis is clinical, and is characterised by fever > 38°C, maternal and fetal tachycardia, uterine tenderness, malodorous amniotic fluid and leukocytosis.

6. A nonreactive NST and absence of fetal breathing movement are the first biophysical manifestations of infection.

7. The predominant risk for patients with PROM between 32 and 36 weeks is chorioamnionitis. Antibiotics must be administered.

8. The main risk in PROM between 28 and 32 weeks is HMD. Administration of corticosteroids and prolongation of gestation are useful.

9. Immediate delivery should be instituted for patients who are in labour, patients with mature fetal lungs, those with fatal fetal malformation, fetal distress, overt or subclinical infection and those with abruptio placentae or cord prolapse.

10. Patients being treated with expectant line of management should be monitored very meticulously for onset of infection.

CHAPTER 17

Prolonged labour

A. BUPATHY

The term prolonged labour includes a wide spectrum of conditions ranging from an apparently harmless prolonged latent phase of labour to the more serious condition of obstructed labour which needs immediate treatment. Prolonged labour may lead to intrauterine asphyxia of the fetus, which may cause permanent neurological damage to the fetus or even fetal death. The mother may suffer from a range of complications like sepsis, injuries to the genital tract and hemorrhage.

The partogram, a graphic documentation of the rate of cervical dilatation and descent of the presenting part in relation to time, is a useful tool for prevention, early detection and proper management of prolonged labour. The incidence of obstructed labour could be reduced significantly if labour is monitored with the help of a partogram.

Objectives

At the end of this chapter, the reader should be able to

❑ Define normal duration of labour.

❑ Define partogram and enumerate its components.

❑ Detect when the partogram reflects prolonged labour.

❑ Appreciate the need for anticipation/early detection of prolonged labour.

❑ Define obstructed labour.

❑ Enumerate the consequences of prolonged labour.

❑ Outline treatment options for each condition.

❑ Refer a case of prolonged labour appropriately.

CLINICAL SCENARIO

A 22-year-old primigravida at term pregnancy, has not delivered after being in labour for 20 hours.

In a primigravida the normal duration of labour should be 12–16 hours; it is much shorter in a multigravida. Labour is said to be prolonged if the woman does not deliver safely within 18 hours.

HISTORY

What additional information should one gather?
Reconfirm the actual duration of labour

This is best done by ascertaining the time when true labour pains started. The characteristics of true labour pains are:

a. True pains start at the back, radiate anteriorly and downwards towards the medial aspect of the thighs.
b. The pain is intermittent, colicky in nature and occurs at regular intervals.
c. The intensity and frequency of pain increases as labour progresses.
d. The onset of pain is associated with blood-stained mucous discharge known as 'show'. Bleeding is due to separation of membranes from the lower segment, and the mucus plug is from the cervical canal.
e. It is associated with cervical changes.

This patient could have suffered from false labour pains when

a. The contractions are irregular.
b. The intensity of pain does not increase.
c. There is no progress of labour by way of cervical dilatation or descent of head.
d. Pain is relieved by sedation.

Review documentation of labour

Documentation may be made as 'notes' or as a partograph. *Partogram is a one page document where the main events of labour are graphically depicted; the rate of cervical dilatation and descent of the presenting part are marked on the vertical axis and the time (in hours) on the horizontal axis.* It shows cervical dilatation in cm and descent of the presenting part in cm in relation to the level of ischial spines which is marked as 'zero' station (Fig. 17.1). The phases of labour are:

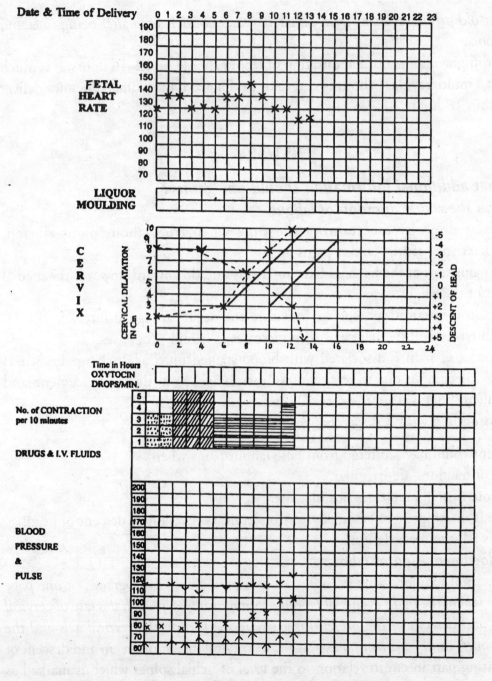

Fig. 17.1 Partogram in normal labour

Date & Time of Admission

Date & Time of Delivery

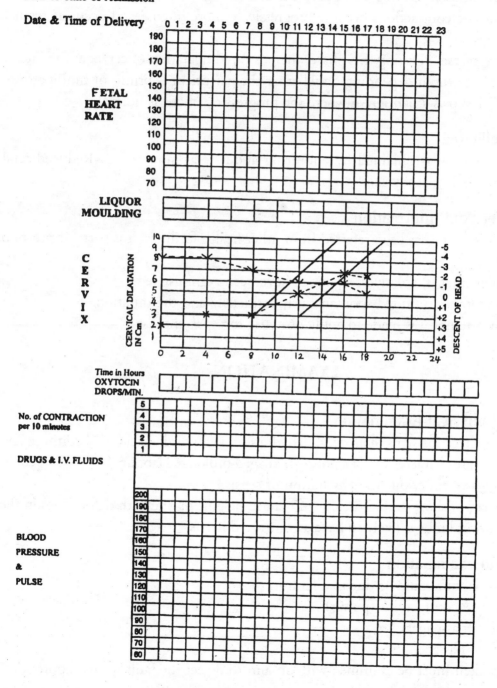

Fig. 17.2 Partogram in prolonged labour

❖ *Latent phase*—During this phase there is negligible cervical dilatation whereas the uterine contractions become progressively more intense and occur at regular intervals.

❖ *Active phase*—During this phase, there is rapid dilatation of cervix at the rate of 1.0–1.5 cm/hour depending on whether the parturient is primi- or multiparous. Fig. 17.1 shows a partogram where the progress of labour is normal.

Fetal wellbeing

This information is obtained by enquiring about fetal movements. Reduced fetal movements reflect asphyxia.

Other relevant information

In case the patient has been referred from other health facilities, it is pertinent to *find out whether*

a. Drugs, that is, sedatives, oxytocics have been administered.
b. Membranes ruptured spontaneously/artificially and the duration.
c. Any attempt was made to apply obstetric forceps/ventouse.

EXAMINATION

General physical examination

One must check for signs of anxiety, dehydration, tachycardia, acidotic breathing and fever which are characteristic of a poorly managed prolonged labour. The patient could be hypotensive either due to dehydration or sepsis.

A woman of short stature (below 145 cm in height) or one with deformities in the spine or lower limbs is likely to have a contracted pelvis.

Obstetric examination

Prolonged labour could be due to a fault in the

a. Uterine contractions (power)
b. Fetus (passenger)
c. Pelvis (passage)

The patient must be examined with an aim to detect the fault so that appropriate corrective measures can be taken.

Abdominal palpation

i)   On palpation, uterine contractions are said to be satisfactory if
  ❖ Three contractions occur in 10 minutes.
  ❖ Each contraction lasts for 40–50 seconds.
  ❖ The uterus is completely relaxed between the contractions.

Assessment of uterine contractions by clinical palpation can be plotted on the partogram.

ii) The lie, presentation and position of the fetus and the estimated fetal weight should be evaluated carefully.

The patient under discussion is a primigravida; occipito posterior position could be a cause for prolonged labour. The need for a long rotation through 135º (Fig. 3.10), a deflexed head and an android type of pelvis delay labour. All these factors may lead to prolonged active phase as determined by cervical dilatation crossing the 'alert' line. Similarly, descent of the head can also be protracted (Fig. 17.2).

Attention is to be paid to abnormal presentations like face, brow and shoulder. In a cephalic presentation, a big baby or malformation like hydrocephalus may be responsible for prolonged labour. In such cases, the head will continue to be felt per abdomen.

The fetal heart should be auscultated and its rate must be counted.

Vaginal examination

A speculum examination may reveal foul-smelling meconium stained liquor or lacerations in the vagina or cervix if there was interference by unskilled personnel.

A bimanual examination must be performed to:

❖ Confirm if patient is in active labour, that is effacement of the cervix, dilatation of 2–3 cm and formation of bag of membranes. If there is no effacement and the dilatation is less than 3 cm, the patient is most probably in the latent phase of labour.

❖ Note if there is edema of the cervix which occurs in prolonged labour due to fault in the passenger or the passage (fetus or pelvis). Under these circumstances, the cervix is not 'well applied' to the presenting part.

❖ See if membranes are present or absent.

❖ Look for caput and moulding, which point towards delay due to cephalopelvic disproportion.

❖ Assess the capacity and architecture of the pelvis.

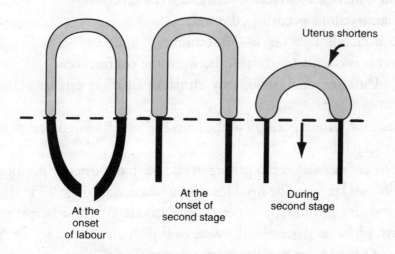

Uterus shortens

At the
onset
of labour

At the
onset of
second stage

During
second stage

Fig. 17.3 a: Change in the upper and lower uterine segments in normal labour

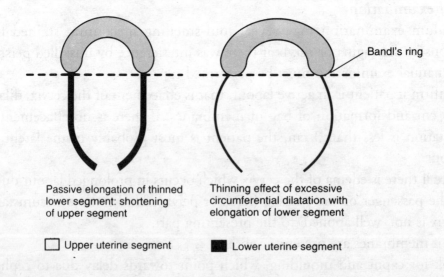

Bandl's ring

Passive elongation of thinned
lower segment: shortening
of upper segment

Thinning effect of excessive
circumferential dilatation with
elongation of lower segment

☐ Upper uterine segment   ■ Lower uterine segment

Fig. 17.3 b. Changes in the upper and lower uterine segments in obstructed labour

Normally the upper segment of the uterus contracts and the lower segment dilates to accommodate the fetus as it is expelled (Fig. 17.3a). However, if there is a fault in the pelvis (for example, contracted pelvis) or a fault in the fetus (for example transverse lie) (Fig. 17.4), the propulsion of the fetus is arrested leading to obstructed labour. Here the upper segment not only contracts, but retracts markedly and consequently the lower segment is stretched and thinned out. If no intervention is instituted, it gives way, resulting in rupture uterus (Fig. 17.3b).

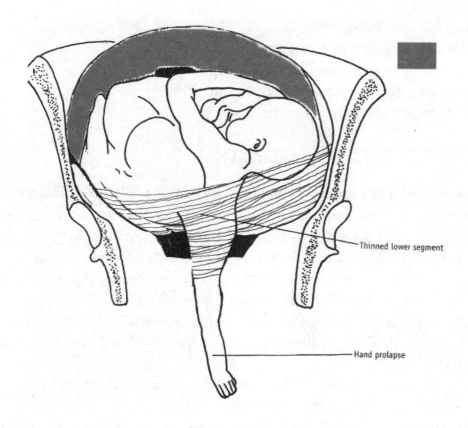

Fig. 17.4 Neglected shoulder presentation

In obstructed labour, the progress of labour comes to a standstill due to mechanical factors in spite of good uterine contractions and, delivery is not possible without assistance. If no intervention is instituted, obstructed labour ends in rupture uterus—a catastrophe, which accounts for 10 per cent of maternal deaths in India.

INVESTIGATIONS

The following investigations must be performed for patients who are admitted with prolonged labour:
1. Hemoglobin
2. Urinalysis for acetone and proteins
3. Serum electrolytes for hyponatremia and hypokalemia
4. Urine and vaginal swab for culture and sensitivity
5. Ultrasonography for abnormal presentation

MANAGEMENT

 How should one proceed to manage a case of prolonged labour?
The information obtained from history and clinical findings and investigations will certainly help to make the diagnosis. The management consists of improving the patient's general condition by allaying apprehension, correcting dehydration, administering antibiotics if the patient is subjected to frequent pelvic examination, or if there is history of prolonged rupture of membranes and evidence of sepsis.

Uterine activity should be augmented if uterine contractions are inadequate and sepsis has not set in. Fetal wellbeing is not compromised when there is uterine hypotonicity.

Operative vaginal delivery in the form of forceps delivery or vaccum extraction is indicated when there is arrest in the second stage of labour (cervical dilatation is 10 cm) due to failure of maternal efforts. Vacuum extraction is particularly indicated in case of deep transverse arrest where midpelvic contraction has been ruled out.

Cesarean section is resorted to if labour is prolonged due to cephalopelvic disproportion, transverse lie, fetopelvic disproportion, persistent mento posterior and brow presentation. In case of deep transverse arrest, cesarean section is indicated if there is midpelvic contraction.

In obstructed labour, cesarean section must be considered if there is abnormal stretching of the lower segment (Bandl's ring) irrespective of the fetal condition. In the absence of signs of threatened rupture and if the fetus is dead, destructive operations like craniotomy are performed to reduce the fetal bulk and deliver it vaginally.

PREVENTION AND EARLY DETECTION

Intelligent antenatal care can detect cases at risk for prolonged/obstructed labour, so that they can be referred to a hospital with facilities for cesarean section.

Inadequate uterine contractions are responsible for prolonged labour in about 60–70 per cent of cases; mechanical factors, as discussed above are responsible in others. If mechanical factors have not been detected during the antenatal period, prolonged labour can be diagnosed early during labour if a partogram is maintained.

The latent phase is said to be prolonged, if it is more than 14 hours in a primigravida and 8 hours in a multigravida. After 'therapeutic rest' with sedation, most women enter into the active phase.

The active phase of labour starts at fully effaced cervix and 3 cm dilatation. The cervical dilatation is plotted on the partogram and an alert line is drawn. The alert line depicts the expected dilatation rate of 1 cm/hour. An action line is then drawn 4 hours parallel and to the right of the alert line.

If the actual cervical dilatation curve stays to the left of the alert line, the progress of labour is normal. If it crosses the alert line, the uterine contractions and the fetopelvic relation must be reassessed. However, if the patient is in a peripheral health facility, she must be referred to a higher health facility. Lastly, if the cervical dilatation crosses the action line, it should be viewed seriously. This shift to the right indicates a need for reassessment and appropriate intervention like correction of dehydration, review by a consultant, augmentation of uterine contraction and operative intervention in the form of cesarean section.

Prolonged labour and its sequelae, both to the mother and her fetus can be reduced significantly by monitoring labour with a partogram.

Key points

1. Labour is said to be prolonged if the woman does not deliver within 18 hours of onset of proper contractions.

2. A partogram is a graphic representation of the rate of cervical dilatation and descent of the presenting part plotted against time in hours.

3. In the latent phase, cervical dilatation is minimal although contractions gradually set in.

4. In the active phase, rapid dilatation of the cervix occurs at the rate of 1 cm/h.

5. Labour may be prolonged due to fault in the power (contraction), passage (bony or soft parts of pelvis) or passenger (fetus).

6. Arrest of progress of labour in spite of effective uterine contractions, due to mechanical factors where delivery is not possible without assistance is known as obstructed labour. It is a preventable condition.

7. Proper recording of partogram helps in early referral and alerts the obstetrician to take appropriate action.

CHAPTER 18

Postpartum hemorrhage

P. Reddi Rani

Postpartum hemorrhage (PPH) is a common and potentially lethal obstetric complication contributing to 28 per cent of maternal mortality. Finding ways to reduce these deaths is a major challenge. The primary aim in the management of PPH should be prevention. Hence, any means of reducing blood loss in the third stage of labour is important. Uterine atony is the most common cause of PPH. Routine administration of oxytocics reduces the risk of PPH by 40 per cent.

Objectives

At the end of this chapter, the reader should be able to

- ❑ Define PPH.
- ❑ Enumerate causes of PPH.
- ❑ Recognise women at risk of developing PPH.
- ❑ Take measures to prevent PPH.
- ❑ Plan the management of PPH.

CLINICAL SCENARIO

A 30-year-old multipara starts bleeding profusely per vaginum immediately following delivery of the baby.

Excessive bleeding into or from the genital tract after delivery of the fetus is defined as PPH. Average blood loss following vaginal delivery and cesarean section is approximately 500 and 1000 ml, respectively. Any higher amount is considered as PPH. But in practice, it is difficult to assess the exact amount of blood loss and therefore a decrease in hematocrit of at least 10 per cent or need for blood transfusion must be considered as criteria of PPH. If the patient is anemic, even a blood loss of < 200 ml, will worsen the general condition of the patient. Also the rate at which blood is lost and the patient's ability to withstand hemorrhage are important.

 ### What are the immediate resuscitatory measures to be taken?

Immediate steps should be taken to control hemorrhage and to combat shock. The most probable cause of PPH in the patient is uterine atony as the patient is multiparous. The mechanism of blood loss in uterine atony is depicted in Fig. 18.1. When the uterus contracts and retracts, blood vessels are occluded and bleeding is arrested (Fig. 18.2). Therefore when faced with this problem, it is best to administer methyl ergometrine 0.2 mg IV or IM, secure an IV line with an 18 gauge cannula and collect blood for cross matching. Preferably, Ringer lactate or any available crystalloid should be infused to replenish the circulatory volume.

 ### How should one manage placental site bleeding?

The uterus is massaged to make it hard. If the bladder is full, it should be catheterised and the patient sedated with 15 mg of morphine IM, ergometrine 0.2 mg is given IV; oxytocin drip with 10–20 units in 500 ml is started and arrangements made for blood transfusion. If the placenta is separated by now, as recognised by true lengthening of the cord, it is delivered by controlled cord traction. If not, the placenta is removed manually under anesthesia.

 ### How should one manage bleeding after delivery of the placenta?

The bleeding, in all probability, is due to uterine atony, and the steps in the management are as described above.

The patient is closely monitored for the following:
* Rise in pulse rate
* Fall in blood pressure
* Urine output
* Further bleeding

The placenta and membranes are examined to make sure they are complete, because retained bits of cotyledons or membranes are the cause of atonicity, leading to continued blood loss. If the uterus is still flabby, methyl ergometrine 0.2 mg and if necessary, 250 μg of 15-methyl PGF$_{2\alpha}$ may be given IM. If the uterus does not contract, both the drugs can be safely repeated. If the bleeding continues in spite of the above measures, the patient should be taken to the operation theatre, and under general anesthesia, one of the following procedures in order of preference is performed to control the hemorrhage.

❖ Bilateral ligation of uterine artery
❖ Bilateral ligation of the internal iliac artery
❖ Hysterectomy

The immediate treatment of PPH is summarised in the flowchart given below.

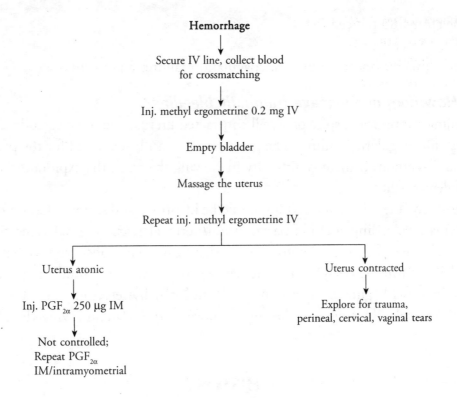

The dose, time of onset, duration of action and side effects of commonly used oxytocics are shown in Table 18.1.

Table 18.1 Uterotonic agents used to control atonic PPH

Agent	Route	Dose	Onset	Duration of action	Side effects
Oxytocin	IV umbilical vein	10–40 U 10 U	30 sec	3 minutes	Water intoxication, hypotension
Methly ergometrine	IV IM	0.2 mg	1 minute 7 minutes	3 hours 3 hours	Nausea, vomiting, hypertension
15 methyl $PGF_{2\alpha}$	IM myometrial	250 µg	15 minutes	8 hours 8 hours	Fever, vomiting diarrhea, asthma

CLASSIFICATION OF PPH

Uterine atony: 80 per cent

Trauma: 15 per cent

Retained placenta and membranes, coagulation failure: 5 per cent

 How does one manage traumatic bleeding?

If bleeding continues in spite of a well contracted uterus, one must exclude associated trauma and coagulation failure. The genital tract must be explored for the presence of any tear/laceration. If there is difficulty in viewing the tract, the exploration is carried out under anesthesia.

Essentially, the source of bleeding should be identified and sutured. Common causes of traumatic bleeding include paraurethral/perineal tears, vaginal lacerations and occasionally, cervical tears. There may be significant blood loss from an episiotomy wound if suturing is delayed. If a hematoma is present, it should be evacuated. If rupture uterus is diagnosed, laparotomy and rent repair/hysterectomy should be resorted to, with the sole objective of *achieving hemostasis quickly* and saving the life of the patient.

HISTORY

Predisposing factors

After delivery of the baby, the muscle fibres of the uterus normally contract so as to occlude the blood vessels and arrest bleeding, thus acting as 'living ligatures' (Fig. 18. 2). However, the muscle fibres fail to contract under the following conditions:

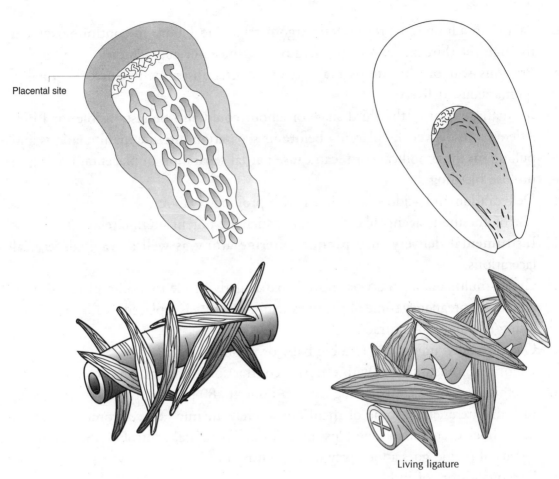

Placental site

Fig. 18.1 Atonic uterus   Fig. 18.2 Well contracted uterus

Living ligature

a. Prolonged labour, especially the second stage, and untimely sedation are responsible for subsequent atony of the uterus.

b. Precipitate labour, where uterus is evacuated so rapidly that it has no time to contract.

c. Antepartum hemorrhage may also be a factor. Whenever there is antepartum hemorrhage, the likelihood of PPH is high because, in the first place, the patients cannot withstand further blood loss. Secondly, if the placenta is on the lower segment, the muscle fibres here cannot occlude the blood vessels; thirdly PPH could be due to coagulation failure so frequently associated with accidental hemorrhage. Therefore, remember that **'if bleeding occurs before delivery, it is very likely to occur after delivery'**.

d. Failure to administer prophylactic ergometrine and failure to continue oxytocin through the third stage, if labour had been induced or augmented.

e. Previous scar on the uterus may give way after instrumental or occasionally, spontaneous, delivery.

f. Mismanagement of the third stage of labour could also be responsible for PPH. Attempts to deliver the placenta before its separation, uterine manipulations and pulling on the umbilical cord, can cause partial separation of placenta, leading to profuse bleeding.

g. Dehydration and acidosis associated with prolonged labour.

h. Use of anesthetic agents like halothane which are potent uterine relaxants.

i. Instrumental delivery may produce uterine atony as well as vaginal/cervical lacerations.

j. Grand multipara, a para 5 or above is particularly prone to atonic PPH, because with every pregnancy some of the uterine musculature is replaced by fibrous tissue, losing its ability to contract.

k. Overdistended uterus due to a big baby or multiple pregnancy.

l. Uterine fibroids interfere with effective contractions of uterine musculature.

m. Anemia could be a contributing cause. About 40–80 per cent of pregnant women in India are anemic; some of them are severely anemic. These women could go into shock even with a blood loss of 200 ml. Therefore, control of anemia in the antenatal period goes a long way in preventing PPH.

n. Previous history of PPH.

Secondary PPH is defined as undue bleeding occurring more than 24 hours after delivery; it usually occurs between the 5th and the 15th day postpartum. It is due to sepsis or retained placental bits and membranes. Treatment must focus on aggressive antibiotic therapy and replacement of blood. Occasionally, surgical treatment may be required.

PREVENTION

PPH can be prevented by active management of the third stage of labour, by administering 0.2 mg ergometrine intravenously at the time of delivery of anterior shoulder which is followed by slow delivery of the fetus taking at least 2–3 minutes. By adopting this measure, the placenta is expected to be delivered following the delivery of the trunk. It reduces not only the duration of the third stage but also the amount of blood loss. Very careful monitoring of the patient is advocated in the third stage, which has been rightly labelled as the 'most treacherous stage of labour' and for an hour later, that is the 'fourth stage' of labour.

During the antenatal period, the following measures can to a great extent, reduce the risk of PPH:

a.   Correction of anemia by giving iron-folic acid prophylaxis and improving nutrition. A pregnant woman should have a hemoglobin of 11 g/dl (WHO 1989).

b.   Referral of cases at risk of PPH for hospital delivery.

Key points

1.   PPH continues to be an important cause of maternal morbidity and mortality.
2.   Uterine atony is the commonest cause of PPH.
3.   Selection of 'at risk' cases for hospital delivery and active management of third stage of labour can effectively reduce the occurrence of PPH.
4.   Methyl ergometrine is a cheap, effective and safe drug and should always be used prophylactically.
5.   Examination of placenta and membranes for completeness is important.
6.   Trauma to the genital tract and coagulation failure as causes of PPH should be looked for if bleeding continues in spite of a well contracted uterus.
7.   Intelligent anticipation, skilled supervision, early diagnosis, as well as prompt and effective treatment will go a long way in reducing maternal mortality due to PPH.

CHAPTER 19

Postpartum collapse

ASHA OUMACHIGUI

RAJEEV SINGH

In an emergency it is strange but nevertheless true, that the more desperate the patient's condition, the more difficult may accurate diagnosis become.

Ian Donald

Postpartum collapse is one of the most dramatic and frightening emergencies. Although, often referred to as 'postpartum collapse', collapse may occur at any point during labour. Intelligent anticipation, early recognition and appropriate management can vastly improve the outcome in most cases.

Objectives

At the end of this chapter, the reader should be able to

- ❏ Enumerate the causes of collapse during intrapartum and postpartum periods.
- ❏ Perform relevant physical examination to determine the cause.
- ❏ Appreciate the need to anticipate collapse.
- ❏ Institute initial resuscitative measures.

CLINICAL SCENARIO

A 25-year-old second gravida collapses suddenly following an operative vaginal delivery.

 What are the measures to be taken at this point of time?

There are several causes for collapse in this patient. One should proceed to institute initial resuscitative measures, which are similar whatever the underlying cause may be. Once the patient is stabilised, the specific cause may be diagnosed and appropriate therapy instituted subsequently.

1. A large bore IV line is started (if the patient does not already have one).
2. Blood is obtained for serum electrolytes, cross match and coagulation studies. Adequate blood should be made available for replacement.
3. The venous return is improved by putting the patient in left lateral position and keeping the legs elevated.
4. Oxygenation is improved by administration of oxygen at the rate of six litres/minute. Ventilation should be assisted if necessary.
5. Even if shock is due to hemorrhage, initial volume replacement could be with crystalloids. An oxytocin drip with 10–20 units/500 ml at 30–40 drops/min is started, once inversion is ruled out.
6. The patient's condition is monitored with regular, and frequent checks on consciousness, pulse, blood pressure, respiratory rate, uterine consistency, vaginal bleeding and urine output. A central venous line (in the absence of DIC) and checks on oxygen saturation are desirable.
7. In a suspected case of amniotic fluid embolism, respiratory passages must be cleared, oxygen administered, and if possible, endotracheal intubation and positive pressure ventilation are employed.

After instituting resuscitative measures, one should proceed to find the cause.

CAUSES

Hemorrhage is the commonest cause of collapse (see also Chapter 18). Often, the blood lost after delivery is not collected and the blood loss is underestimated. There are instances where a slow trickle from an unsutured episiotomy can cost the patient more than 500 ml of blood loss. Lastly, the blood could remain collected in the uterine cavity with very little seen outside. These situations must be detected and adequate blood should be replaced.

Only a minority of patients collapse during or after labour in the absence of excessive hemorrhage. Collapse in such patient could be attributed to two groups of conditions.

1. Blood is lost but it is not revealed.
2. Shock is due to other factors.

One should proceed to search for the bleeding site. In most cases, the sites are within the uterine body, the peritoneal cavity and retroperitoneal spaces. A difficult instrumental delivery, a previous scar in the uterus due to cesarean section, and unrecognised uterine rupture can be antecedents to bleeding into the peritoneal cavity. This can be detected by the presence of free fluid. The blood could also collect within the leaves of broad ligament and in the retroperitoneal spaces. A broad ligament hematoma if large enough, can be detected clinically. Ultrasonography is certainly useful.

An examination under anesthesia could help to detect uterine inversion, or uterine rupture. The presence of paravaginal hematoma or cervical tear can be detected by a vaginal examination. Appropriate surgical intervention should be performed.

Other causes of collapse are :

❖ *Concealed accidental hemorrhage* (see Chapter 12).

❖ *Acute inversion* is often the result of using Crede's manoeuvre and cord traction to deliver the placenta in an atonic uterus.

❖ *Ruptured uterus,* particularly if the rupture is on the posterior aspect of the uterus.

❖ *Amniotic fluid embolism* may occur late in labour or in the immediate postpartum period. It is usually preceded by strong uterine contractions. It is characterised by acute pulmonary embarassment. Treatment by endotracheal intubation and intermittent positive pressure ventilation must be instituted instantly.

❖ *Adrenocortical insufficiency* leads to collapse in cases of pre-eclampsia/eclampsia after delivery. These cases respond to administration of corticosteroids.

❖ *Endotoxic shock,* often encountered in septic abortion, may also be seen in severe chorioamnionitis following prolonged rupture of membranes.

It is mandatory to monitor the patient continuously and ensure that she is stabilised. Plasma fibrinogen and fibrin degradation products (FDP) need to be evaluated as coagulation failure occurs in all the conditions discussed above.

COINCIDENTAL CAUSES OF COLLAPSE

Sometimes, a pregnant woman or one who has just delivered is likely to collapse, due to non-obstetric factors. While instituting resuscitative measures and searching for obstetric factors, it is advisable to consider the following conditions that could lead to collapse:

❖ Acute cardiac failure
❖ Pulmonary embolism
❖ Anesthetic accidents
❖ Reaction to drugs
❖ Previous corticosteroid therapy

Awareness of the existence of medical or obstetric complications, the control of these diseases, prevention of anemia, maintaining hydration during labour and a careful management of the third stage of labour contribute significantly to the reduction of risk of postpartum collapse.

Key points

1. Faced with postpartum collapse, the first step is to institute resuscitative measures.

2. Postpartum hemorrhage is the commonest cause of collapse. Bleeding should be controlled and blood should be replaced.

3. If there is no revealed hemorrhage, efforts should be made to determine obstetric causes of collapse and appropriate treatment should be instituted.

4. One must suspect amniotic fluid embolism based on obstetric history, and vigorous resuscitative measures should be instituted immediately.

5. A parturient may suffer from coincidental diseases that may lead to collapse.

6. Intelligent anticipation, not losing one's nerve in an emergency, early recognition and appropriate management, significantly reduce maternal morbidity and mortality.

CHAPTER 20

Fever in the postpartum period

ASHA OUMACHIGUI

Fever in the postpartum period is usually due to infection of the genital tract. In the last 25 years, there has been a dramatic fall in the incidence and severity of puerperal infection. However, in developing countries its incidence continues to be high; infection ranks with hemorrhage and eclampsia as one of the three prime 'killers' in obstetrics. In India, infection accounts for 20 per cent of all maternal deaths. Appropriate management of pregnancy and labour, judicious use of antimicrobials and above all the practice of asepsis and antisepsis are essential in order to reduce maternal morbidity and mortality caused by puerperal infection.

Objectives

At the end of this chapter, the reader should be able to

❑ Define puerperal pyrexia.

❑ Explain why a woman is prone to develop infection after delivery.

❑ Elicit clinical features suggestive of important causes of fever in the postpartum period.

❑ Select relevant investigations and interpret the results.

❑ Enumerate the common pathogens responsible for postpartum infection.

❑ Institute rational antimicrobial and other therapy as required.

❑ Appreciate the fact that puerperal infection can be prevented.

❑ Take measures to prevent the occurrence of puerperal infection.

CLINICAL SCENARIO

A para 2 has delivered a baby seven days ago. She presents with history of high fever and foul-smelling vaginal discharge.

HISTORY

 What questions should be asked to gain a better understanding of the case?

The patient must be interrogated about the *time of onset of fever after delivery*. The development of fever 24 hours after delivery and within 10 days should alert one to the presence of infection. **Puerperal pyrexia is defined as temperature of 38°C (100.4°F) or more, on any two occasions in the first ten days postpartum,** recorded by an oral thermometer by a standard technique. This definition is not entirely satisfactory as some patients with infection may either have low grade fever or no fever at all. However, the fever could be due to infection of the genital tract or other infection that may occur during the puerperium as at other times. Although fever and infection are not synonymous, puerperal infection is a notifiable disease in many countries and the presence of fever is accepted as a valid criterion.

Foul-smelling discharge per vaginum refers to foul-smelling lochia and points to endometritis. The amount of discharge is less and is purulent or serosanguinous when associated with infection of cervical, vaginal and episiotomy wounds.

1. Irrespective of the presence or absence of foul-smelling vaginal discharge, one must enquire about *burning micturition and increased frequency of micturition*. Pain in the renal angle is suggestive of pyelonephritis.

2. *Pain and swelling of lower limbs* and difficulty in walking alerts one about the possibility of deep vein thrombosis, and this should be remembered while performing physical examination.

3. It would be worthwhile to probe into the events during the antenatal period to find out if the patient had any foci of infection. Presence of urinary tract infection predisposes to recurrence in the postpartum period.

4. There is a need to elicit information regarding certain events in the intrapartum period which promote infection. These are (a) premature rupture of membranes, (b) prolonged labour, (c) frequent vaginal examinations, particularly when performed with disregard to asepsis and antisepsis and (d) internal electronic fetal monitoring.

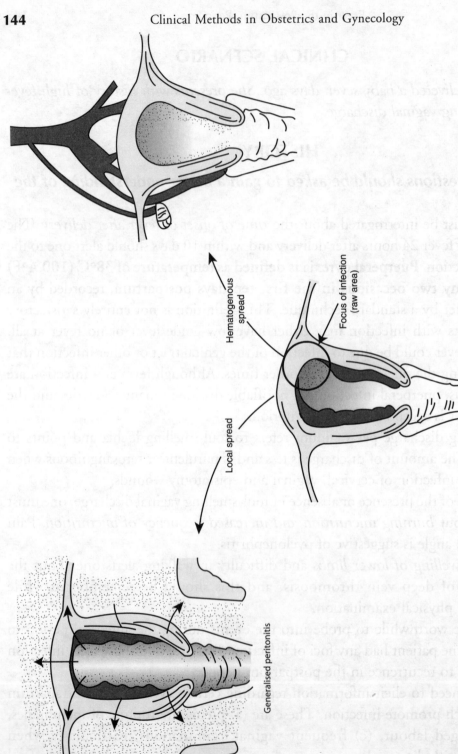

Hematogenous spread

Focus of infection (raw area)

Ascending infection

Local spread

Generalised peritonitis

Fig. 20.1 Mode of spread of puerperal endometritis

5. In a patient suspected to have postpartum infection, one must enquire about the nature of delivery. Infection is relatively uncommon (2.6 per cent) following a vaginal delivery. **However, there is always the potential to develop infection, as the area of the placental bed denuded of endometrial lining is equivalent to a wound elsewhere in the body.** The infection can spread to other systems (Fig. 20.1).

6. If a *cesarean section* has been performed, the risk of developing uterine infection due to a wound on the uterus and abdominal wall is almost 50 per cent. It would be prudent to conclude that a woman who has undergone a cesarean section has 20 times more chance of developing infection as compared to a woman who has had a vaginal delivery.

PHYSICAL EXAMINATION

While performing physical examination, particular attention should be paid to the general condition. The patient is likely to be toxic when the infection is very severe. High spiking fever is also a characteristic of mastitis, breast abscess and pyelonephritis. Low grade fever is associated with deep vein thrombosis.

Tachycardia is usually recorded in all cases of infection. Hypotension occurs in Gram negative septicemia.

Make a note of the degree of pallor as some of these patients are likely to have had postpartum hemorrhage.

Examination of the breasts may reveal uniform swelling and tenderness if the breasts are engorged. Breast engorgement is caused by a sudden increase in the flow of milk leading to distension of lactiferous ducts localised to one of the quadrants. Redness of the skin and fluctuation point towards breast abscess. It is essential to look for retracted/cracked nipples which may be the cause of breast engorgement.

In most cases, abdominal palpation is unremarkable except for a subinvoluted and tender uterus. If the patient had a cesarean section, one should carefully look for induration, wound disruption and infection. Features of pelvic or generalised peritonitis are abdominal distension, tenderness, guarding and rigidity.

Inspection of external genitalia, could reveal infection of the episiotomy wound or perineal tear. A gentle speculum examination should be performed in order to detect lacerations of the vagina, and the cervix, and the source of the abnormal discharge or foul-smelling lochia.

A bimanual examination is useful for confirming subinvolution and tenderness of the uterus, collection of pus in the pouch of Douglas and the presence of paravaginal hematoma.

MANAGEMENT

At this stage it is worthwhile to pause and consider the possible causes, as listed below:

✤ Endometritis
✤ UTI
✤ Breast engorgement/abscess
✤ Deep vein thrombosis
✤ Enteric fever
✤ Viral fever
✤ Malaria
✤ *Endometritis (endomyometritis)*—The presence of risk factors for infection during the intranatal period are premature rupture of membranes and cesarean section. Foul-smelling discharge is characteristic of endometritis. Peritonitis could further complicate the condition. If the woman presents with an acute abdomen, a surgical consultation should be obtained. Once a clinical diagnosis is reached, empirical antibiotic therapy should be started. The infection being polymicrobial, antibiotics effective against most of these organisms should be chosen. A combination of ampicillin, gentamicin and metronidazole is not only effective in most cases of endometritis, but is also cost effective; it can be started once the vaginal swab and urine are sent for bacterial culture.

Dosage: ampicillin 500 mg IV/6 hourly
            gentamicin 1.5 mg/kg IV/8 hourly
            metronidazole 500 mg IV/8 hourly

✤ *In urinary tract infection,* apart from the clinical features, a microscopic examination showing 10 pus cells/HPF is helpful in confirming the diagnosis. Ampicillin should be started while awaiting the results of bacterial culture. Most patients (85–90 per cent) will respond to this treatment within 48–72 hours in both endometritis and urinary tract infection. If there is no response, the case should be reviewed, further investigations conducted, and management changed, if necessary.

On reviewing the clinical features, if they are still suggestive of endometritis or urinary tract infection, one must check the results of bacterial culture and sensitivity and take a blood sample for culture; changing over to β lactam antibiotics like cefoxitin, cefotetan, cefotaxime, extended spectrum penicillin and clavulinic acid along with ampicillin/amoxycillin is advisable, depending on the sensitivity of the organism.

Common pathogens responsible for postpartum infection

Aerobes
- Group A streptococci
- Enterococci
- Gram negative bacteria: E. coli, Klebsiella, Proteus

Anerobes
- Peptostreptococci
- Peptococcus sp
- Fidus
- *Bacteroides fragilis*

Others
- Mycoplasma hominis
- Chlamydia trachomatis

If peritonitis persists, abdominal ultrasonography will help to detect a pelvic abscess or very rarely, a forgotten swab, if the patient had a cesarean section. In about 15 per cent of patients, there may be other causes for fever.

Breast engorgement, as discussed earlier could be associated with fever. The treatment consists of:

Analgesics

Breast support

Expression of breast milk manually; injection of 10 units of oxytocin prior to expression is helpful.

Correction of retracted/cracked nipple

Encouraging the mother to breast feed the child

Antibiotics are not required.

- *Breast abscess and mastitis* represent serious complications. A breast abscess should be incised under general anesthesia and drained, and penicillin group of antibiotics should be administered. The mother can continue to feed the baby from the other breast.

❖ *Deep vein thrombosis*

If there is pain and swelling particularly of one lower limb, associated with low grade fever and tachycardia, one must seriously consider the possibility of deep vein thrombosis. Tenderness of calf muscles on firm palpation clinically points to the diagnosis; it is confirmed with the use of Doppler ultrasonography. Appropriate treatment is instituted.

Initial management

Bed rest

Analgesics

Heparin

Long term management

Warfarin/Heparin

Dosage

Heparin: Initially, 10,000 units SC 8 hourly or 20,000 units SC 12 hourly

(Aim: to prolong PTT by 1.5–2.5 times)

Later 7,500–10,000 units SC 12 hourly without monitoring

Warfarin: sufficient to prolong PT by 1.5–1.8 times

❖ *Respiratory problems* are likely to occur among patients who have been administered general anesthesia for cesarean section/operative vaginal delivery. A proper history, thorough examination of the respiratory system and X-ray of the chest will confirm the diagnosis. Appropriate therapy must be instituted according to the type of problem.

Persistent fever, not responding to antibiotics or the absence of features of endometritis, should make one investigate for pyrexia due to diseases like enteric fever, viral fever and malaria. In all such cases, a peripheral smear for malarial parasite and Widal test are worth performing.

PREVENTION OF POSTPARTUM INFECTION

In a majority of cases, the postpartum fever is due to infection of the denuded area at the placental site and infection of wounds. It must be remembered that a woman delivering spontaneously with an intact genital tract is prone to infection because of the denuded area at the placental site. Therefore, infection in the postpartum period is largely preventable by strict adherence to aseptic and antiseptic precautions. Simple measures like patient's hygiene, detection and treatment of infection during the antenatal period, using a clean place and sterile instruments for delivery, are of immense value.

During the lying-in period, one should be watchful with regard to the woman's complaints of abdominal pain, abnormal discharge, presence of tachycardia, pyrexia and the nature of lochia. Check if there is difficulty in breast feeding. Wounds, if present, must be examined for evidence of infection. Intervention should be instituted immediately with prudent use of antibiotics and other measures. At cesarean section, surgical antibiotic prophylaxis must be employed; a single dose of a broad spectrum antibiotic administered with clamping of cord, significantly reduces the risk of postoperative infective morbidity.

There is certainly much to be said about the importance of counselling a pregnant mother about personal hygiene at all times, particularly about the cleanliness of perineum after delivery and exclusive breast feeding. **These simple preventive measures along with rational use of antibiotics can reduce the risk of postpartum morbidity and mortality.**

Key points

1. Puerperal pyrexia is most often due to infection of the urogenital tract.
2. Endometritis presents as foul-smelling vaginal discharge and UTI as dysuria and increased frequency.
3. PROM, prolonged labour, frequent vaginal examinations disregarding asepsis and antisepsis, and internal electronic fetal monitoring predispose to endometritis.
4. When a cesarean section is performed, the chances of developing infection increase by 20 times compared to a vaginal delivery.
5. Ampicillin, gentamicin and metronidazole are the initial drugs of choice. They should be changed, if required, depending on the clinical response in 48 hours and antibiograms of the cultures.
6. Lack of response may be due to other medical problems like malaria.
7. Regular antenatal care, adequate intranatal care and strict adherence to aseptic and antiseptic measures will reduce the incidence of puerperal fever.
8. Deep vein thrombosis is managed with bed rest, analgesics and heparin.
9. Breast engorgement can be prevented by correction of retracted/cracked nipples during the antenatal period, and by encouraging breast feeding.

CHAPTER 21

Postpartum depression

R. CHANDRASEKARAN

During the postpartum period, 85 per cent of women experience some type of mood disturbances. Though these are mild and transient in nature, in some women it can assume a serious proportion. It is important to recognise and treat these persistent mood disturbances as it otherwise places both the mother and infant at risk. Postpartum disorders remain underdiagnosed because of nonrecognition of these disturbances as specific disorders by the existing classification system. Although to be classified as a postpartum disorder, the onset of the episode is specified as within four or six weeks of the postpartum period, in clinical practice, many depressive episodes have an insidious onset and begin four to five months after delivery.

Objectives

At the end of this chapter, the reader should be able to
- ❏ Describe the clinical features of postpartum 'blues' and depression.
- ❏ Discuss the differential diagnosis of postpartum depression.
- ❏ Appreciate the role of various causative factors in postpartum psychiatric disorders.
- ❏ Demonstrate familiarity with the treatment approaches available for postpartum psychiatric disorders.

CLINICAL SCENARIO

A 28-year-old primigravida with no personal or family history of mood disorders had an uneventful pregnancy and delivery. Fifteen days after delivery, she reported feeling anxious and depressed. Over the next 10 days, these symptoms progressed. She had interrupted sleep. She lost her appetite, her feelings of sadness deepened and persisted throughout the day. She started thinking of ending her life though she never made an attempt to do so. She became withdrawn and was found to be slow in her activities. She started caring less and less for her child which ultimately ended in total neglect of the child. Physical examination did not reveal any abnormality.

HISTORY

 ### What questions should be asked to gain a better understanding of the case?

One must enquire whether the patient had delirium, which is usually characterised by alteration in sensorium, memory and perceptual disturbances. One should look for evidence of infections. History should also focus on symptoms of hypothyroidism. Information should be obtained regarding treatment with medication such as antihypertensives.

An attempt should be made to elicit whether there are marked shifts in the clinical presentation. For example, the syndrome may change rapidly from one of confusion to one with prominent delusions and hallucinations.

Like other medical illnesses, efforts are made to identify the role of psychosocial stressors in this case. Poor family support, marital discord, and disruption of the mother's previous lifestyle are some factors which may contribute to the exacerbation of postpartum psychiatric disorders.

DIAGNOSIS

This patient suffers from postpartum depression. Unlike the postpartum 'blues' or postpartum psychosis which have a rapid onset, postpartum depression has an insidious onset. The mood symptoms are more sustained.

The course of the illness is typically prolonged. No organic factors are identified. Depressive features dominate the clinical picture.

TYPES OF POSTPARTUM PSYCHIATRIC SYNDROMES

These are of three major types:
* Postpartum blues
* Postpartum depression
* Postpartum psychosis

Postpartum blues

This is usually not considered a disorder. It occurs in 50–80 per cent of women, and major symptoms of depression are not evident. It generally appears 3–4 days postpartum and resolves spontaneously within a week. The condition is characterised by crying spells, irritability, rapid mood shifts and broken sleep. Stressful events during pregnancy, marital dissatisfaction, inadequate social support, past history of mood disorders and depression during pregnancy are some of the risk factors associated with postpartum blues.

Postpartum depression

This condition develops more insidiously, and occurs in 10–15 per cent of postpartum women. Sadness, irritability, inability to experience pleasure, insomnia, reduced energy and suicidal ideation are frequently reported. Somatic symptoms may dominate the clinical picture. In its severe form, postpartum depression results in severe dysfunction.

Postpartum psychosis

In the majority, the symptoms appear within the first two weeks of delivery and a second peak may be seen 1–3 months after delivery. Confusion, memory impairment, irritability and anxiety coupled with psychomotor agitation are some of the symptoms experienced. Intrusive thoughts, usually about harming the infant, are not uncommon. Paranoid delusions and auditory hallucinations are also reported. Blatant disinterest towards the child may also be seen. There is a mercurial changeability of the symptoms. A brief period of elation characterised by incessant talking, increased energy may shift rapidly to profound sadness. Lucid intervals followed by florid psychotic behaviour are common. Though the clinical picture resembles an affective disorder, delirium is often found to coexist with this disorder.

CAUSES

Endocrine factors

The postpartum period is characterised by a rapid shift in the hormonal environment. The sudden and drastic decline in serum estrogen and progesterone levels following delivery may be responsible for postpartum psychiatric disorders. In addition, the acceleratory decline in cortisol level following delivery is also implicated. A high incidence of abnormalities in thyroid function tests are relatively common during the postpartum period. Overt clinical signs of hypothyroidism are present in 10 per cent of women following childbirth and the incidence surpasses the number observed in nonpregnant controls. Addition of thyroxine to psychotropic medication may bring about rapid alleviation of psychiatric symptoms in such instances. Estrogen and prednisolone in the treatment of postpartum disorders have met with moderate success. However, these are not used regularly in clinical practice. There may also be various degrees of pituitary dysfunction following delivery.

Psychosocial factors

Stressful events during pregnancy or near the time of delivery, marital dissatisfaction and inadequate social support are some of the psychosocial variables implicated in postpartum disorders.

TREATMENT STRATEGIES

Pharmacological intervention

In *postpartum depression* with symptoms of agitation and anxiety, sedative anti-depressants like imipramine and amitryptiline are appropriate. The starting dose is 50 mg and the dose may be increased by 25–50 mg, every second or third day up to 150–200 mg per day or until adverse effects occur. Upward titration should be done cautiously if the individual is medically compromised. The patient should be given the maximum dose for 4–6 weeks. Adjunctive use of a benzodiazepine (such as clonazepam, lorazepam) is recommended if anxiety symptoms are prominent. Sleep, energy and appetite are the first to improve. Improvement in mood and depressive cognition takes a long time. If no improvement occurs, the tricyclic drug is augmented with lithium or a different antidepressant is tried. Though the single bedtime dosage of a tricyclic drug is often followed, it is for the physician to decide on the dosage schedule, depending on the side effects. If the depression is associated with compulsive features, treatment with serotonin specific reuptake inhibitors like fluoxetine (20–80 mg/day) and sertraline (50–200 mg/day) may be used. However, side effects like agitation are to be closely monitored. In case of severe depression associated with high suicidal intent, electroconvulsive therapy is the treatment of choice. When prescribing antidepressants, the physician may recommend stopping breast feeding. Associated disorders like hypothyroidism and Cushing syndrome have to be treated separately.

Postpartum blues is a mild and transitory mood syndrome. Reassurance, observation and occasionally a short-acting sedative are the primary interventions. Those with a previous history of mood disorder should be closely monitored for signs of postpartum depression.

Postpartum psychosis merits hospitalisation because of the level of dysfunction and the grave risk of infanticide. Lithium or other mood-stabilising medications are helpful in controlling the affective syndrome. Antipsychotic drugs like risperidone (2–8 mg/day) may be used to control hallucinations and delusions. In severe and refractory cases, electroconvulsive therapy is indicated.

Psychosocial intervention
It is useful to emphasise the biologic aspects of postpartum illness, as many women might not have experienced a mental illness before. This helps in alleviating feelings of failure and guilt. It is also important to convey the message that postpartum illness has a good prognosis. Support groups and education are known to be beneficial to postpartum women during recovery.

BARRIERS TO DIAGNOSIS

The postpartum illness in general begins 3–4 days after parturition. Most patients are discharged within 48 hours after delivery and hence the symptoms of postpartum psychiatric disorders are not identified immediately, thereby making the mothers vulnerable. Stigma is another barrier to an early consultation and patients conceal the problems out of shame and guilt. Though postpartum blues are self-remitting disorders, occasionally it can be a prodrome of a more severe postpartum depression. If this is not recognised, patient will be deprived of treatment with antidepressant drugs.

Key points

1. Postpartum blues is a self-limiting, relatively mild mood syndrome experienced by 30–80 per cent of all postpartum women. The onset is usually on day 3 or 4 of parturition and the symptoms remit within two weeks. Reassurance is all that is needed in the majority of the cases.

2. Postpartum depression develops in 10–20 per cent of women after delivery. The onset is generally insidious and the mood symptoms are more sustained.

3. Postpartum psychosis is relatively rare (0.1–0.2 per cent) and the clinical picture though resembling an affective disorder, is often associated with delirium and confusion.

4. The sudden decline in serum progesterone, estrogen and cortisol levels following delivery are implicated in the pathogenesis of postpartum psychiatric disorders. Abnormalities in thyroid function are relatively common during the postpartum period.

5. Postpartum depression is treated with either tricyclic antidepressants or serotonin specific reuptake inhibitors. Electroconvulsive therapy is indicated in severe cases of depression associated with high suicidal risk.

6. Psychosocial interventions include education and use of support groups.

CHAPTER 22

Examination of a normal newborn

B. Vishnu Bhat

A normal newborn is one who is delivered at term and weighs more than 2500 g, is without any asphyxia, birth injury or congenital malformations, and is able to take oral feeds with active sucking. It is essential that any abnormality in the baby is diagnosed early in order to give appropriate treatment.

Objectives

At the end of this chapter, the reader should be able to

- ❑ Enlist the physical findings in a normal newborn.
- ❑ Appreciate the need to examine a newborn thoroughly.
- ❑ Recognise features that deviate from the normal.
- ❑ Identify sick babies and refer them appropriately.

EVALUATION

General

- ❖ Weight should be more than 2500 g but less than 3700 g; average birth weight varies from region to region. It may vary from 2800 to 3000 g in the developing countries.
- ❖ Length may vary from 47–52 cm.
- ❖ Head circumference measures 32–35 cm and it is usually 3 cm more than chest circumference.
- ❖ Skin temperature is 36–36.5ºC.

❖ Respiration—periodic breathing without cyanosis or bradycardia at a rate of 40–60/min is normal during the neonatal period.

❖ Heart rate is 120–160/min. Examination of the heart may reveal a soft systolic murmur which could be functional. However, organic heart disease may exist even without an audible murmur.

❖ Blood pressure should be— Systolic pressure 40–60 mm Hg
Diastolic pressure 25–40 mm Hg

Skin

❖ Cyanosis of extremities and sometimes of lips (acrocyanosis) is common during the first few days. Presence of central cyanosis (mucus membranes) except immediately after birth should suggest a serious disorder.

❖ Physiological jaundice may be visible on the third day and usually disappears by 7–10 days of life. Visible jaundice in a newborn indicates a serum bilirubin of > 5 mg/dl. Appearance of icterus during the first 24 hours of life or involvement of palms and soles is suggestive of severe hyperbilirubinemia and may require exchange transfusion.

❖ Plethora/purple colour indicates polycythemia and is seen more often in growth retarded babies, infants of diabetic mothers and when there is feto-fetal or materno-fetal transfusion.

❖ Pallor may be due to blood loss, sepsis or shock and needs immediate correction.

❖ Harlequin colour changes where the baby may have pink and pale halves due to vasomotor instability.

❖ Mongolian spots are bluish patches usually seen over the buttocks and back. They are due to melanocyte deposits and usually disappear by six months to two years of age.

❖ Hemangioma usually disappears by the time the child is 2 years old. However, large hemangiomas may be associated with thrombocytopenia. Intracranial lesions may be associated when they occur over the face (Sturge–Weber syndrome).

❖ Milia are whitish papular lesions, the size of a pin-head, and are usually seen all over the face. These sebaceous retention cysts disappear within 2–3 weeks.

❖ Erythema toxicum usually appears after two days of life. They are mostly papular, but can be macular or vesicular with erythema all around and disappear within seven days.

Head

❖ Moulding of skull occurs during the birth process; it is normal and gets corrected by 2–3 days of life.

❖ Edema of the skin and the subcutaneous tissue over the presenting parts is known as caput succedaneum and lasts for 2–3 days. Cephalhematoma is due to the collection of blood under the periosteum; unlike caput succedaneum, it is limited by the suture lines, may be associated with skull fracture and takes 6–8 weeks to resolve.

❖ The anterior and posterior fontanelles are usually open at birth. The posterior fontanelle closes by 2–4 months while the anterior one remains open for 12–18 months.

Face

❖ Eyes—Subconjunctival hemorrhage at birth can be normal. Blue sclera may be associated with osteogenesis imperfecta. Downward slant of the eyes with Brushfield iris indicates Down syndrome.

❖ Depressed bridge of the nose and hyperteleorism are associated with chromosomal defects.

Mouth

❖ Epstein pearls—They are small pin-head size retention cysts seen over the junction of the hard and soft palates and disappear after a few days.

❖ The retention cysts over the floor of mouth are known as ranula and will resolve spontaneously.

❖ Natal teeth are occasionally present. Since they are loose, there is risk of aspiration; they may also injure the mother's nipple while sucking. Therefore, these teeth may have to be extracted.

Neck

The neck appears relatively short in the newborn. One should look for swellings such as cystic hygroma or thyroglossal cyst. Presence of webbing of the neck with widely spaced nipples and increased carrying angle at the elbow are indicative of Turner syndrome.

Chest

❖ Enlargement of breasts due to maternal hormones is normal during 3–7 days of life. This is known as *mastitis neonatorum*. The breasts should not be squeezed to remove the 'milk' since this will predispose to breast abscess by opening up the lactiferous tubules.

❖ Functional cardiac murmurs (grade III or less) may be heard. Presence of thrill, cyanosis or cardiac failure indicate organic heart disease.

Abdomen

❖ Liver (2–3 cm) and spleen (tip) are normally palpable, but markedly enlarged liver or spleen and easily palpable kidney require investigation.

❖ There are two arteries and one vein visible over the umbilical stump. A single umbilical artery is associated with internal congenital anomalies.

Genitalia

Male

Testes are at the bottom of the scrotum in term babies. Undescended and abnormally placed testes are to be recorded and evaluated later if persistent. *Phimosis* is normal during this period but the meatus can be viewed on retraction of the prepuce in more than 85 per cent of male newborns.

Female

Vaginal discharge and bleeding during the first 3–7 days of life is normal due to withdrawal effect of maternal hormones. Mucosal tag may be present at introitus. Marked clitoral hypertrophy suggests congenital adrenal hyperplasia.

Extremities

One should look for polydactyly, foot deformities (talipes), and congenital dislocation of the hip. Adducted position of the hip with creases over the medial side of the thigh indicates congenital dislocation of the hip.

Back and spine

The back should be examined for meningocele or meningomyelocele. Spina bifida occulta may be suspected by the presence of tuft of hair, dimple or swelling over the lower spine.

Passage of urine and meconium

New born babies usually pass urine within the first 24 hours. Often urine is passed during delivery. If the baby is normal without any abdominal distension, increased feeding will usually cause micturition.

Meconium is normally passed during the first 12–24 hours. When there is delay, a soft rubber catheter may be passed into the rectum for confirming rectal patency. **The finger or tip of a thermometer should not be introduced into the rectum for testing patency!** Passage of meconium could be delayed in case of prematurity, mucus or meconium plug, Hirschsprung's disease (congenital megacolon), meconium ileus, or hypothyroidism. Low enema is useful in resolving meconium plug.

MANAGEMENT OF THE NORMAL NEWBORN

❖ *Temperature support*—The newborn should be dried and covered after birth to prevent heat loss. It may take 12–24 hours for temperature to stabilise.
❖ *Cord care*—The umbilical stump should be cleaned with spirit and kept dry to prevent colonisation with infective bacteria. Local application of antiseptic lotions like triple dye is not required.
❖ The eyes should be cleaned with wet sterile cotton. There is no need to instil silver nitrate or antibiotic drops into the conjunctival sac routinely, except when there is increased incidence of conjunctivitis in the locality, especially due to gonococci. When prophylaxis is necessary, a single local application of tetracycline or erythromycin ointment is advised; silver nitrate application may cause chemical conjunctivitis.
❖ Breast feeding should be initiated as early as possible and should not be delayed for more than 3 hours. Preterm and low birth weight babies in particular need to be fed early. A normal healthy baby should receive 7–8 feeds in the first few days.

DANGER SIGNS IN THE NEWBORN

The baby needs to be evaluated when the following signs are present:
❖ Reduced activity or hypotonic
❖ Poor sucking
❖ Persistent vomiting/bile-stained vomiting

❖ Abdominal distension
❖ Baby is cold or warm to touch
❖ Jaundice occurring on the first day or involving the extremities or lasting for more than two weeks
❖ Pallor may indicate anemia or shock
❖ Bleeding
❖ Convulsions

Babies with these features may be referred to a higher centre for management.

Key points

1. Birth weight, length and head circumference of Indian babies are less than that observed in developed countries.
2. Features like mongolian spot, toxic erythema, milia, and Epstein pearls are normal findings.
3. Babies usually pass urine and meconium within 24 hours of delivery.
4. Breast milk is the ideal feed for the baby.
5. Identification of sick babies and appropriate referral is essential for better outcome.

CHAPTER 23

The infant who does not breathe at birth

B. Vishnu Bhat

Perinatal asphyxia results from inadequate oxygenation of the fetus and is biochemically associated with hypoxemia, hypercapnia and acidosis. It is usually indicated by an Apgar score of ≤ 3/10 at 1 minute and ≤ 6/10 at 5 minutes.

However, in preterm babies, Apgar score and blood gases do not always correlate. Apnea with severe bradycardia lasting for more than 5 minutes after birth, is associated with a high mortality and neurological handicap among the survivors.

Objectives

At the end of this chapter, the reader should be able to

❑ Define perinatal asphyxia.
❑ Differentiate primary from secondary apnea.
❑ Identify risk factors for asphyxia.
❑ Evaluate the Apgar score of a baby.
❑ Enlist ABCs of resuscitation.
❑ Resuscitate an asphyxiated baby.
❑ List the steps of resuscitation.

CLINICAL SCENARIO

A primigravida at term comes with ruptured membrane for ten hours and draining meconium-stained liquor. She had been administered pethidine two hours earlier. At birth, the baby is pale, limp and gasping.

How does one differentiate between primary and secondary apnea?

Apnea at birth can be classified as primary or secondary. Primary apnea is the initial apnea following rapid respiration in response to hypoxic insult. Secondary apnea follows slow irregular breathing after primary apnea. It is associated with hypotension and pallor and always requires positive pressure ventilation. It is not possible to diagnose the type of apnea at birth. Since delay in initiating breathing will make subsequent resuscitation difficult, leading to brain damage, one has to treat all cases of apnea at birth as secondary apnea.

 What are the risk factors for hypoxia in the newborn?

❖ **Preterm or post-term delivery**—A preterm baby has poor respiratory effort and can aspirate easily. A post-term baby may have intrauterine hypoxia due to placental insufficiency. It may also suffer from meconium aspiration.

❖ **Multiple pregnancy**—There may be delay in the delivery of the subsequent babies.

❖ **Hydramnios**—The baby is likely to have upper intestinal obstruction or open neural tube defects.

❖ **Rh isoimmunisation**—There may be anemia and hydrops in the fetus.

❖ **Congenital malformations**—Major malformations may lead to asphyxia and difficult resuscitation.

❖ **Maternal sedation**—Sedative drugs administered to the mother may result in respiratory depression in the baby.

❖ **Operative deliveries**—These may be undertaken for nonprogression of labour or for fetal distress. There is risk of birth injuries, if instrumental vaginal delivery has been performed.

❖ **Infants of diabetic mothers**—They are at increased risk for malformations and may be delivered preterm. Due to macrosomia, they may suffer from birth injuries.

❖ **Prolonged rupture of membrane**—This may predispose to infection in the baby.

❖ **Antepartum hemorrhage**—Blood loss may lead to hypotension and hypoxia.

❖ **Malpresentation and obstructed labour**—Difficult delivery may lead to birth injuries and hypoxia.

 What are the important findings to be sought?

❖ **Apnea or slow irregular breathing** – It will lead to hypoxia in the baby.

❖ **Cyanosis**—Presence of central cyanosis indicates poor oxygenisation, but peripheral cyanosis is usually present during the first few days of life.

❖ **Pallor** – This may result from blood loss or myocardial damage due to hypoxia.

Severe and prolonged asphyxia may lead to multiorgan failure (respiratory, cardiac, central nervous system and renal).

Table 23.1 Apgar scoring

Feature	Score		
	0	1	2
Appearance (A)	Pale or central cyanosis	Peripheral cyanosis	Pink
Heart rate/pulse (P)	Nil	<100	>100
Grimace reflex (G)	Nil	Poor response	Good response (sneezing and crying)
Activity/Tone (A)	Flabby/hypotonic	Minimal flexion of limbs	Good flexion with active movement
Respiration (R)	Nil	Slow and irregular	Regular

The Apgar score is useful in objectively evaluating the baby and is done at one, five and ten minutes and every five minutes thereafter till the baby is normal. Since the Apgar score is first done only at 1 minute, it should not be used for initiating resuscitation. However, it can be helpful in evaluating the response of the baby to resuscitation. Initial evaluation is based on three signs—respiration, heart rate and colour. The resuscitation efforts should be tailored to suit the individual needs of the baby.

ABCS OF RESUSCITATION

The ABCs of resuscitation are *airway* establishment, *breathing* initiation, and *circulation* maintenance.

 What are the steps involved in resuscitation?

The steps can be divided into

❖ Initial steps
❖ Bag and mask ventilation
❖ Endotracheal intubation
❖ Chest compression
❖ Medication

Initial steps in resuscitation

* The baby is placed under a radiant warmer, head down 10–15° with mild extension of the neck.
* The baby is dried and the wet cloth is removed.
* The mouth is suctioned first and then the nostrils. If the nose is suctioned first, it will stimulate respiration and allow the secretion from the nasopharynx to be aspirated.
* Tactile stimulation is provided if the baby is apneic or is breathing in a shallow manner. Two accepted methods for tactile stimulation are, flicking or tapping the foot and rubbing the back. *Do not* slap the baby, press over the chest or abdomen, dilate the anal sphincter or sprinkle hot and cold water. The majority of babies will require only the initial steps of resuscitation.

Use of bag and mask in resuscitation

Indications for bag and mask ventilation include apnea and heart rate < 100/min, and persisting cyanosis.

Volume of the bag used for neonatal resuscitation should not be more than 750 ml. Newborns should be resuscitated with 90–100 per cent oxygen. Press the bag with the fingers and not with the palm. The baby should be initially ventilated with a pressure of 30–40 cm H_2O while subsequent breathing will require only 15–20 cm H_2O. However, a diseased lung may require as much as 20–40 cm H_2O pressure. The baby should be ventilated at a rate of 40–60/min. The baby should be placed supine with mild extension of the neck. The mask is held tightly with the thumb and index finger, with the other fingers steadying the chin. The mask should cover the nose and mouth but not the eyes. If the baby's chest fails to rise, check for:

* Tear in the bag or mask
* Size of the mask (ideal-sized mask should cover the nose, mouth and chin but not the eyes)
* Secretions or vomitus in the pharynx
* Position of the neck (mild extension)
* Adequacy of pressure

Indications for endotracheal intubation

* Thick meconium-stained liquor
* Diaphragmatic hernia should be suspected when there is scaphoid abdomen. Such

a baby should not be ventilated with bag and mask, since it may result in distension of intestine and cardiorespiratory compromise.
* Poor response to bag and mask
* Need for prolonged ventilation

Indications for cardiac compression
Indications for cardiac compression include a heart rate of < 60/min or 60–80/min and not increasing with positive pressure ventilation.

Technique of chest compression
Compress the lower third of sternum, that is, the area just below the horizontal line joining the nipples. Do not press over the xiphoid process since it may cause a tear in the liver.

There are two methods for cardiac compression—two finger method and thumb method. In the two finger technique, the middle finger and the index or ring fingers are used for compression while the palm of the other hand supports the back of the child. The thumbs of both hands are used for compressing and the torso of hands supports the back in thumb method. However, the area for compression, the rate and depth remain the same in both the techniques. The rate of compression is about 120/min and the depth is about 1–1.5 cm.

USE OF DRUGS

The following drugs may be used depending on the indications.

Epinephrine
Dose: 0.1–0.3 ml/kg of 1 in 10,000 solution
Indication: Heart rate < 80/min, after ventilating with 100 per cent oxygen for 15 seconds
Route: IV or intratracheal

Naloxone
Dose: 0.2 mg/kg
Indication: Respiratory depression in a baby delivered within 6 hours of mother receiving a narcotic.
Route: IV or intratracheal

Sodium bicarbonate

Dose: 2 meq/kg of 4.2% solution

Indication: Documented acidosis

Route: IV; administer over 5–10 minutes

Volume expander

O negative blood, plasma, albumin, normal saline or Ringer lactate

Dose: 10 ml/kg over 5–10 minutes

Indication: Evidence of hypovolemia

Dopamine

Amount: Initially 5 µg/kg/min, and increased to 20 µg/kg/min, if necessary. The amount of dopamine to be added in milligrams to 100 ml of fluid is calculated by the formula

(6 x weight in kg x dose in µg/kg/min) ÷ desired amount of fluid in ml/hour

Indication: Persisting hypotension after volume expansion

COMPLICATIONS

❖ Pneumothorax

❖ Injury to face

❖ Injury to trachea and esophagus

❖ Hypoxic ischemic encephalopathy

❖ Myocardial, brain and renal damage in severe asphyxia

The treatment is outlined below:

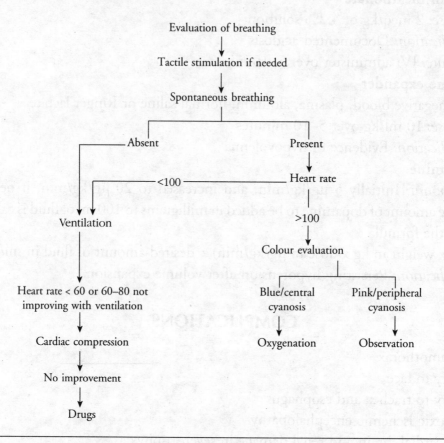

Key points

1. Resuscitation at birth is an emergency procedure.
2. Every apnea at birth should be treated as secondary apnea.
3. The majority of babies will require only initial steps of resuscitation.
4. Babies with suspected diaphragmatic hernia should not be given bag and mask ventilation.
5. Hypoxic babies will require evaluation and long-term follow up.

CHAPTER 24

The yellow baby

B. VISHNU BHAT

Mild yellow discolouration of a baby's body during the first few days of life is a common occurrence. The majority of infants recover spontaneously. Due to the risk of brain damage from high levels of bilirubin, early recognition, evaluation and treatment are indicated.

Objectives

At the end of this chapter, the reader should be able to

- ❑ Define neonatal jaundice.
- ❑ Enlist the common causes of jaundice.
- ❑ Differentiate physiological from pathological jaundice.
- ❑ Evaluate clinically the severity of icterus.
- ❑ Conduct appropriate investigations.
- ❑ List the indications for phototherapy and exchange transfusion.

CLINICAL SCENARIO

A mother with O +ve blood group delivers a baby at term with A +ve group. The baby develops jaundice involving the extremities, on the second day of life.

Visually noticeable yellow discolouration of the skin and mucous membrane usually indicates a serum bilirubin of more than 5 mg/dl.

HISTORY

 What questions should be asked to gain a better understanding of the case?

Time of *onset* and *duration* should be ascertained. Almost 65 per cent of term and 75 per cent of preterm babies develop icterus during the first few days of life.

Physiological jaundice may be due to many reasons such as:

✤ Increased red blood cell breakdown and production of bilirubin
✤ Poor uptake of bilirubin by the liver because of immaturity of acceptor proteins
✤ Deficiency of glucuronyl transferase enzyme
✤ Increased enterohepatic circulation due to paucity of gut flora.

History of jaundice in the previous baby indicates blood group incompatibility. The subsequent babies will have similar severity of jaundice in ABO incompatibility. Usually an A group baby born to an O group mother will have increased risk of jaundice. ABO blood group incompatibility is much more common than Rh hemolytic disease.

In Rh incompatibility, the first baby is not affected since the mother has no natural antibodies. The risk of neonatal jaundice increases in subsequent pregnancies. Sometimes minor incompatibilities may also cause significant jaundice.

✤ Infections, both intrauterine or postnatal, can cause jaundice.
✤ Exaggerated physiological jaundice may occur due to prematurity, maternal consumption of drugs, extravascular blood collection like cephalhematoma or extensive ecchymosis.
✤ Other hemolytic disorders like G6PD deficiency, pyruvate kinase deficiency, hereditary spherocytosis and hemolytic anemias may be responsible for jaundice in the newborn.

INDICATORS OF PATHOLOGICAL JAUNDICE

The following criteria point towards pathological jaundice:

✤ Visible jaundice on the first day of life
✤ Serum bilirubin level of more than 12 mg/dl, in term, and >15 mg/dl in preterm babies. One should be careful when the baby has very low birth weight; even low levels of bilirubin could be dangerous.
✤ Direct bilirubin is more than 2 mg/dl

* Rate of rise is >5 mg/dl per 24 hours
* Presence of anemia or hepatosplenomegaly
* Reticulocyte count >8 per cent
* Jaundice persisting for >2 weeks

EVALUATION

* Antenatal screening of parents' blood groups for incompatibility is important. This will help in identifying babies who are likely to develop significant icterus.
* Clinical evaluation for severity of jaundice should be done under bright light. The icterus has a cephalocaudal progression depending on the intensity. When only the face and mucous membrane are yellow, the bilirubin level will be approximately 5 mg/dl. When the chest and upper abdomen are involved it will be 10 mg/dl and involvement of lower abdomen and thighs suggests 15 mg/dl. If there is involvement of palms and soles, the level will be more than 20 mg/dl.
* One should check for presence of anemia and hepatosplenomegaly indicative of hemolysis.
* Poor feeding, lethargy and irritability suggest sepsis or kernicterus if the jaundice is very severe.

INVESTIGATIONS

* One should determine the blood group of the mother and baby. It is helpful in detecting blood group incompatibility.
* Direct Coomb's test in cord blood is done in order to identify the presence of antibodies. It will be positive when the mother is already sensitised.
* Reticulocyte count more than 15 per cent indicates severe hemolysis.
* Serum bilirubin should be monitored serially for appropriate management.
* Peripheral smear examination is necessary. Presence of increased number of nucleated red blood cells and spherocytes suggests ABO incompatibility.
* Blood culture, white cell count and other septic screening tests should be conducted if infection is suspected.

MANAGEMENT

 How should one proceed to treat this infant?

Phototherapy is generally used when the serum bilirubin level is more than 5 mg/dl below the exchange transfusion level. When the skin is exposed to light, there is photoisomerisation and photo-oxidation of bilirubin into water-soluble compounds which can be excreted through bile and urine. White, blue or green light can be used. The wavelength of the light should be in the range of 400–500 nm. Intensity of the light recommended is 4–5 mw/cm^2 body surface area. Normally, phototherapy can reduce the serum bilirubin by 2–4 mg/dl/24 hours. It can bring down the exchange transfusion rate by 70–80 per cent. Phototherapy is discontinued when there is no further risk from hyperbilirubinemia. Since direct bilirubin is water-soluble, there is no role for phototherapy in direct hyperbilirubinemia.

Side effects of phototherapy

Unstable temperature, skin rashes, diarrhea, damage to the eyes, dehydration, hemolysis and gonadal damage are some of the side effects of phototherapy.

Exchange transfusion should be initiated if cord blood bilirubin is >5 mg/dl, hemoglobin <12 g/dl, reticulocyte count >15 per cent, serum bilirubin >10 mg/dl on the first day, 15 mg/dl in the 48 hours after birth, or 20 mg/dl any time after birth.

In low birth weight babies, the upper limit of safe bilirubin level in mg/dl is obtained by dividing the weight of the baby in g by 100.

RH HEMOLYTIC DISEASE

This occurs when the mother is Rh –ve and the baby is Rh +ve from a positive father. The mother usually gets sensitised after the delivery of an Rh +ve baby. Since there are no natural anti-Rh antibodies in the mother, the first baby is not affected. The mother can, in rare cases, become sensitised during the later months of pregnancy when the placenta becomes more permeable to fetal red cells.

Rh hemolytic disease is not common. The reasons for this are:

❖ Only 5–7 per cent Indians are Rh negative.
❖ There is 25 per cent chance of having an Rh negative baby when the father is heterozygous.

❖ The quantum of feto-maternal transfusion may be small or the mother may not produce enough antibodies.

❖ If there is coexisting ABO incompatibility, it will give relative protection against Rh disease, since the fetal cells will be destroyed in maternal circulation.

❖ Where consanguineous marriages are common, both parents may have similar Rh type.

❖ Administration of Rh immunoglobulin to the mother within 72 hours of delivering an Rh +ve baby, gives protection against development of antibodies in her.

MANAGEMENT OF A BABY BORN TO AN RH NEGATIVE MOTHER

When the mother is Rh −ve, the father's blood group should be determined. If the father is also negative, there is no Rh incompatibility. When the father is Rh +ve, perform an indirect Coomb test in the maternal blood in order to find out whether the mother is sensitised. When Coomb's test is negative in the mother, a normal outcome for the baby can be expected.

In a baby born of an Rh −ve mother, check the baby's blood group and Rh type, direct Coomb status, bilirubin and hemoglobin levels. The baby should be examined for anemia, hepatosplenomegaly and edema. When they are present, exchange transfusion should be undertaken. A severely affected fetus may be stillborn or delivered with hydrops fetalis.

ABO HEMOLYTIC DISORDER

This usually occurs when the mother has O blood group and the baby has A or B. Since A group is more antigenic, O–A incompatibility causes more severe icterus in the baby. Unlike Rh hemolytic disease, there is no need for prior sensitisation, and the first baby may be affected since antibodies are present naturally. Levels of serum bilirubin and hemoglobin are related to the amount of hemolysis. Direct Coomb's test is weakly positive.

Peripheral blood smear shows increased reticulocytes and microspherocytes. It is difficult to differentiate hereditary spherocytosis from ABO hemolytic disease in the newborn period since the peripheral smear picture will be similar.

The jaundice is usually mild and may not require any treatment. When there is significant icterus, phototherapy is initiated. Exchange transfusion is undertaken in severe cases. Since ABO incompatibility is more common, exchange transfusion is done in neonatal units more often for this condition than for Rh hemolytic disease.

 What is kernicterus?

Kernicterus or bilirubin encephalopathy is caused by the deposition of bilirubin in the brain stem. The damage caused is not reversible and the baby will have chorcoatheroid cerebral palsy with deafness. In the initial phase the baby will have reduced activity and poor sucking. Later, the baby will develop convulsions and oculogenic crisis. Proper management of hyperbilirubinemia can prevent this condition.

Key points

1. Early recognition, evaluation and treatment of jaundice are essential for preventing bilirubin encephalopathy (kernicterus).
2. ABO incompatibility is more common, but Rh hemolytic disease is more severe.
3. Rh hemolytic disease increases in severity in subsequent pregnancies unlike ABO incompatibility.
4. Phototherapy can reduce the exchange transfusion rate by 70–80 per cent.
5. Jaundice manifesting on the first day, involving extremities, or associated with anemia or hepatosplenomegaly, is pathological.

CHAPTER 25

The baby with convulsions

B. Vishnu Bhat

A baby with convulsions may be suffering from seizure disorder or it may just be jittery. Seizure disorder is an acute central nervous system emergency requiring immediate therapy while jitteriness is usually innocuous. The incidence of convulsion varies from 2 to 3 per cent among newborn babies.

Convulsion is defined as abnormal movements of the body due to sudden increase in cerebral discharge, with altered level of consciousness.

Objectives

At the end of this chapter, the reader should be able to

- ❑ Define neonatal convulsions.
- ❑ Enumerate the types of convulsions.
- ❑ Differentiate seizure from jitteriness.
- ❑ List the common causes of convulsions.
- ❑ Identify the babies at risk.
- ❑ Conduct appropriate investigation.
- ❑ Suggest a treatment plan for neonatal convulsion.

CLINICAL SCENARIO

A full term female baby was delivered after meconium staining of liquor was noted. The baby had an Apgar score of 2/10 at 1 minute, 5/10 at 5 minutes and 7/10 at 10 minutes. The baby developed respiratory distress at birth. At eight hours of age, the baby was noted to have tonic movements of the limbs with rolling up of eyeballs.

HISTORY

 What are the risk factors one should look for?

One should check for:

* **Perinatal asphyxia:** it is the single most important cause of neonatal convulsions.
* There may be **intracranial bleed** and injury due to birth trauma.
* **Metabolic abnormalities** are common among small for gestational age babies, preterm and postterms, babies of diabetic mothers, and those who sustained birth asphyxia. Common abnormalities include hypocalcemia, hypoglycemia and hypomagnesemia.
* **Hyponatremia** may develop in babies of mothers who received dextrose without saline.
* **Pyridoxine dependency or deficiency** should be looked for.
* **Hyperbilirubinemia** causing kernicterus may develop after 3–5 days of birth. It can be prevented by exchange transfusion.
* **Intracranial infections** are generally caused by bacteria and often manifest three days after birth.
* Withdrawal effect of maternal medications especially opiates.
* Inadvertent injection of local anesthesia into fetal scalp vein.
* Congenital malformations of the central nervous system.

TYPES OF CONVULSIONS

Almost 40–50 per cent of convulsions during the neonatal period are subtle or subclinical. The subclinical seizure is indicated by:

* Staring spells
* Jerky movement of the eyes
* Prolonged blinking
* Lip smacking or chewing movements
* Cycling movement of the limbs
* Attacks of irregular respiration, cyanosis or apnea
* Unexplained paroxysmal stiffness, fisting or flaccidity

A manifest convulsion could be of the following types:

* Focal clonic

* Focal tonic
* Multifocal
* Myoclonic—Myoclonic convulsion has the worst outcome since it is often associated with underlying brain abnormality. Generalised convulsions are uncommon during the neonatal period.

FEATURES OF JITTERINESS IN THE NEWBORN

* Movements are fine and tremulous
* Irregular in frequency
* Can be stopped by holding the limb or flexing the joint
* No change in gaze or level of consciousness
* Absent during sleep
* Normal electroencephalograph (EEG)

INVESTIGATIONS

Estimation of blood sugar, serum calcium, magnesium and serum electrolytes should be done. Meningitis is excluded by blood culture and lumbar puncture in relevant cases. Cranial ultrasound, MRI, EEG and CT scan are helpful in localising intracranial lesions in resistant cases and when convulsion recurs.

MANAGEMENT

 How should one proceed to treat a baby with convulsions?

The following drugs are given sequentially:

* 10% glucose 4–6 ml/kg and 6–8 mg/kg min maintenance is administered.
* 10% calcium gluconate 1.5–2 ml/kg (15–20 mg/kg of elemental calcium) is given intravenously; if convulsions persist give 80–200 mg/kg of elemental calcium as maintenance.
* Pyridoxine 100 mg IV is given in pyridoxine dependency or deficiency (50–100 mg/day as maintenance).
* If hypocalcemia persists, hypomagnesemia is probable and $MgSO_4$ 50 per cent solution 0.2 ml/kg IM is administered.

❖ Phenobarbitone 20 mg/kg is given intravenously as loading dose (3–5 mg/kg as maintenance).

❖ If convulsions still persist, phenytoin 20 mg/kg as loading dose is administered IV (5 mg/kg maintenance).

❖ If convulsions continue to persist, paraldehyde 0.1–0.3 ml/kg is given by deep intramuscular or rectal route, or the baby is put on diazepam/midazolam as slow infusion.

Most convulsions in newborns are of short duration. Since metabolic disorders often cause seizures in the newborn, anti-convulsants are usually not needed. Recurrent attacks, presence of neurological signs, family history of convulsions and evidence of brain damage will warrant long term administration of anti-convulsants.

Key points

1. High risk babies should be monitored for convulsions.
2. Subtle convulsions account for 40–50 per cent of neonatal convulsions.
3. Convulsions should be differentiated from jitteriness.
4. Perinatal hypoxia is the most common cause for convulsions in developing countries.
5. Metabolic abnormalities are an important cause.
6. Although convulsions may occur among 2–3 per cent of babies, only a few of them need long term anti-convulsants.

CHAPTER 26

The septic baby

B. VISHNU BHAT

Sepsis or infection of the baby by the invading microorganisms is one of the important and common causes of neonatal morbidity and mortality. The infection may be acquired transplacentally, during delivery or later from the personnel or the environment. The incidence varies from 15–20 per thousand live births.

Objectives

At the end of this chapter, the reader should be able to

- ☐ Define neonatal sepsis.
- ☐ Identify risk factors for neonatal infection.
- ☐ Enlist the common causative microorganism.
- ☐ Enumerate the signs and symptoms.
- ☐ Conduct relevant investigation.
- ☐ Outline appropriate management.
- ☐ List the steps in preventing neonatal sepsis.

CLINICAL SCENARIO

A mother at 34 weeks of gestation delivered a baby with two days history of leaking per vaginum. The baby cried immediately after birth and tolerated tube feeds. On the third postnatal day, the baby developed fever with reduced activity.

Neonatal sepsis is characterised by systemic signs associated with bacteremia. It can be of early onset (during first seven days of life) or late onset (after seven days) type. The baby presented above was a preterm baby, and was more over, born following leaking per vaginum for two days.

HISTORY

❖ *Premature delivery* increases the risk of sepsis. Preterm babies are in a compromised state. They have poor barrier against infection and are likely to undergo more procedures.

❖ *Prolonged rupture of membranes*—The chances of a baby developing infection are markedly increased when the membranes rupture more than 24 hours before delivery.

Other factors

❖ *Birth asphyxia* supresses the immune system.

❖ *Birth injuries* may result in open wounds which can easily get infected.

❖ *Chorioamnionitis*—Infection of the amniotic fluid can result in infection of the baby.

❖ *Maternal infections*—Viral, treponemal and toxoplasma infections can affect the fetus.

❖ The infection can be acquired from personnel or *contaminated environment.*

❖ Lack of aseptic and antiseptic precautions during procedures can cause infection.

❖ Any IV cannula placed for intravenous access may cause infection.

❖ *Congenital malformations* can predispose to infection.

❖ Male babies are at 2–3 times higher risk for infection probably because of a single X chromosome.

CAUSES

The agents responsible for neonatal infections are shown in Table 26.1.

SIGNS OF NEONATAL INFECTION

❖ *Lethargy and poor feeding* are the early common features that suggest sepsis in a baby.

Table 26.1 Causative agents in neonatal infections

Early onset < 7 days		Late onset > 7 days
Intrauterine	**Postnatal**	
Toxoplasma	Group B streptococcus	Staphylococcus
Cytomegalovirus	E. coli	Klebsiella
Rubella	Chlamydia	Pseudomonas
Treponema pallidum	H. influenzae	Acinetobacter
Herpes simplex		
Hepatitis B		
Listeria		

❖ *Temperature instability* is seen. Usually, hypothermia is noted among preterms and hyperthermia in term babies.

❖ *Tachypnea, respiratory distress or apnea* may suggest associated bronchopneumonia.

❖ *Rashes in the form of petechiae or ecchymosis* indicate intravascular coagulation or thrombocytopenia.

❖ When there is *abdominal distension,* the baby may be suffering from ileus or necrotising enterocolitis.

❖ *Unexplained jaundice* may be present (see Chapter 24).

❖ *Mottling or marbling of the skin* indicates vasomotor instability.

❖ *Altered sensorium, convulsions and bulging fontanelle* may be present when meningitis is associated.

INVESTIGATIONS

The babies who are preterm, delivered after prolonged rupture of membranes, born to mothers with known infection, sustained severe birth asphyxia or invasive procedures, need to be screened for sepsis.

❖ Absolute white cell count may be 5,000–30,000/mm³. A count of less than 5,000 or more than 30,000 with a neutrophilic shift to left may suggest infection. The band cell to neutrophil ratio exceeds 0.2 with presence of toxic granulations.

❖ The erythrocyte sedimentation rate in the newborn equals the postnatal age in days plus three in mm per hour. Increased ESR is a non-specific finding suggestive of infection.

❖ When the C-reactive protein level is increased to more than 4 mg/dl, it is suggestive of infection.

Band cell count, micro ESR and CRP level, together can have a sensitivity and specificity of 90–95 per cent in diagnosing neonatal sepsis. They are used as initial screening tests.

❖ *Blood culture*—Isolation of the causative agent from the blood is a definitive sign of sepsis, but it is positive in two-thirds of the cases.

❖ *Urine culture*—The causative organism can be identified from urine culture in a significant number of cases.

❖ *Lumbar puncture* may be necessary. Neonatal sepsis is associated with meningitis in 30 per cent of cases. The prognosis is poor and duration of therapy is longer when meningitis is present.

❖ *Counterimmunoelectrophoresis* can be used for rapid diagnosis of sepsis. Since it is based on the presence of bacterial antigens, the test can be positive even after the administration of antibiotics.

❖ *Blood sugar* should be closely monitored for associated hypoglycemia. When there is bleeding, investigations for disseminated intravascular coagulation should be done. Blood gas analysis should be undertaken when there is significant respiratory distress.

MANAGEMENT

How does one proceed to manage the above case?

❖ General measures
    a. Maintaining proper temperature
    b. Adequate nutrition and hydration
    c. Respiratory and cardiovascular support with close monitoring of respiratory rate, heart rate and blood pressure

❖ Specific steps consist mainly of medications, varying according to the type of infection. Initial choice of antibiotics should be based on the experience in the particular unit. Usually, a combination of ampicillin with gentamicin is used. The therapy can be modified based on the response and the culture reports. If the newborn was only a suspected case and the investigations do not confirm sepsis, the therapy can be stopped after 72 hours. Babies with positive culture should be treated for 10–14 days. Septicemia associated with meningitis should be given 2–3 weeks therapy. Osteomyelitis and septic arthritis will require 3–4 weeks treatment.

Other modes of therapy like exchange transfusion, granulocyte transfusion, immunoglobulin administration, fibronectin therapy have been tried but the results are not consistently encouraging.

The steps involved in the management of babies with risk factors are outlined below.

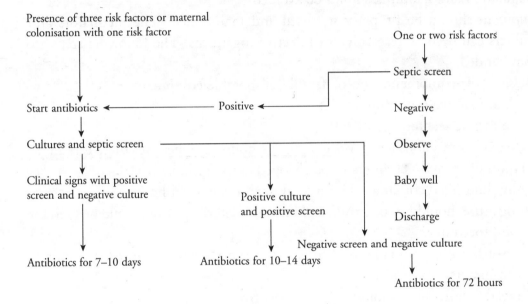

PROGNOSIS

The mortality from neonatal sepsis may vary from 30 to 50 per cent depending on the type of organism, birth weight and gestational age of the baby, and the presence of other complicating factors. Babies with severe septicemia, especially those with meningitis, may suffer from permanent sequelae and neurological handicap.

STEPS TO PREVENT INFECTION

❧ *Washing hands* is the single most important and effective procedure for controlling infection. Hands should be washed with soap and disinfectants for three minutes before entry into the nursery, and every eight hours thereafter. Before handling each baby, hands should be washed. Surgical scrubbing is essential before every procedure.

❖ Since overcrowding increases the risk for infection, there should be *1–2 metres gap between the cots.*

❖ *Particular care should be taken of the skin, cord and eye*—The intact skin and the normal flora are natural protective barriers against infection. Unnecessary manipulation and handling should be avoided.

❖ *Equipment* should be properly sterilised and maintained. The incubators and nebulisers can become reservoirs for infective organisms. The following steps are recommended:

✦ Use sterile equipments and preferably, disposable equipment.

✦ Avoid invasive procedures.

✦ Use aseptic techniques.

✦ Change intravenous access once in 48–72 hours, or whenever there is redness.

✦ Humidifiers and nebulisers to be changed every 24 hours.

✦ Any fluid-filled container should be flushed once in 24 hours.

❖ *Nursing attire* should not be a source of infection. Sterile gowns should be used for invasive procedures.

✦ Personal clothing and unscrubbed parts of the body should not come in contact with infants.

✦ Infected individuals should be kept away from babies.

❖ *Cohorting* is an important infection control method for limiting outbreak of an infection.

✦ Babies with same infection or organisms should be grouped.

✦ Infected babies should be cared for by separate nurses.

✦ After all the cohorts are discharged, the area should be cleaned and disinfected.

Nosocomial infections are the leading causes of neonatal morbidity and mortality. Strict hand washing, periodic screening of personnel and adherence to aseptic techniques are critical for minimising infections in nurseries.

Key points

1. Sepsis may occur in 15–20 per 1,000 live births.
2. Signs of sepsis may be subtle. It is important to have a high index of suspicion.
3. High-risk babies should be screened for infection.
4. Babies with three or more risk factors need treatment pending investigation results.
5. Antibiotic administration should be based on nursery experience.
6. Mortality may be 30–40 per cent.
7. Proper hand washing, avoiding invasive procedures and indwelling catheters, use of disposables and aseptic precautions will reduce the incidence of sepsis.

CHAPTER 27

White discharge per vaginum

S. HABEEBULLAH

White discharge is a common complaint among women presenting in the gynecologic clinic. In adults, a small amount of vaginal discharge is normal. *Leukorrhea*, which means an excess of normal vaginal discharge, is mucoid, non-purulent, non-offensive, and is not associated with irritation. Sometimes this term is used loosely for any white discharge per vaginum.

Objectives

At the end of this chapter, the reader should be able to

- ❑ Recognise physiological vaginal discharge.
- ❑ Enumerate the causes of abnormal vaginal discharge.
- ❑ Enumerate the common organisms producing vaginitis.
- ❑ Recognise specific infections of the vagina and cervix from the symptoms and signs.
- ❑ Appreciate that some women are likely to predominantly experience itching of the vulva.
- ❑ Choose tests to confirm diagnosis.
- ❑ Outline therapy for abnormal white discharge.
- ❑ Counsel those with physiological discharge.

CLINICAL SCENARIO

A 40-year-old multiparous woman presents with complaints of vaginal discharge associated with itching.

HISTORY

 What questions need to be asked to gain a better understanding of the case?

❖ *Age* should be ascertained. The patient under discussion is 40 years old. In the reproductive age group, infections, especially vaginitis, account for 90 per cent of cases of white discharge.

Physiological discharge, due to increase in circulating estrogens or progesterone, may manifest in the newborn and at puberty. In adults, white discharge is found to occur pre-menstrually, at midcycle and during pregnancy; it is also brought on by sexual excitation. In the postmenopausal woman, the possibility of senile vaginitis, senile endometritis and uterovaginal prolapse should be considered.

❖ Sudden *onset* suggests infection, particularly if it follows unprotected coitus and the individual has multiple sexual partners. Chronic onset suggests physiological discharge; one should also consider the possibilities of chronic cervicitis or erosion.

❖ *The amount and type of discharge* should be questioned. The need to wear a sanitary napkin suggests excessive discharge. It is excessive and frothy in case of trichomonal vaginitis whereas in monilial vaginitis, the discharge tends to be scanty, thick and curdy.

❖ *Colour* should be noted. A curdy white discharge suggests monilial infection, whereas greenish yellow discharge is present in trichomoniasis. Purulent discharge is characteristic of pyogenic infection. A dark brown or red colour suggests presence of blood which is common in neoplasms (such as cancer cervix).

❖ *Odour* is indicative. Foul-smelling discharge is present in trichomonal vaginitis, gardnerella vaginitis and in cancer cervix.

❖ *Pruritus must be enquired into.* Itching is commonly associated with both trichomonal and monilial vaginitis. Gonococcal infection causes 'soreness' of the vulva. Moniliasis also tends to involve the vulva and is said to cause vulvovaginitis.

In some women, particularly those who are in the peri- or postmenopausal age group, pruritus is a predominant symptom. There may or may not be a history of white discharge. In the absence of vaginal infections, they are said to be suffering from 'pruritus vulvae'.

Pruritus vulvae may be a part of generalised pruritus with systemic disorders like diabetes mellitus, hepatic disorders with jaundice or chronic renal failure. In older women, vulvar epithelial dystrophies (example, leucoplakia) cause pruritus. Other skin diseases such as psoriasis, scabies, and tinea can affect the vulva.

Urinary incontinence and infestation with Enterobius vermicularis or Trichuris trichura can often be related to itching of vulva particularly in children and adolescents.

❖ *Other symptoms*—Vaginal discharge due to infection tends to be associated with dysuria and lower abdominal pain. Diabetes mellitus is strongly associated with monilial vulvovaginitis and pruritus vulvae. Pregnancy, systemic antibiotic therapy, chronic anemia, oral contraceptives and immunosuppressive drugs like corticosteroids favour moniliasis.

❖ *Male partner*—History suggestive of genital infection in the male partner or multiple sexual partners point to sexually transmitted infection.

❖ *Other information*—One must check about the use of vaginal tampons and spermicides. If the symptom is essentially pruritus, contact dermatitis due to cosmetics, deodorants and douches should be excluded.

PHYSICAL EXAMINATION

❖ The general condition of the patient with reference to nutritional status and anemia should be noted.

❖ The vulva, perineum and thighs should be inspected for signs of excoriation, scratch marks, ulcers and general hygiene. The vulva should also be inspected carefully for the presence of red and white lesions. Urethral meatus and Bartholin glands should be observed and palpated; normally Bartholin glands are not palpable.

❖ Before performing speculum examination the patient must be asked to strain, to rule out genital prolapse.

❖ Speculum examination should be performed to note the characteristics of the discharge such as colour, quantity and odour. In moniliasis, a thick, curdy white discharge is seen adhering to the vaginal wall, which on removal reveals inflamed vagina. In trichomoniasis, the appearance of the vagina is described as 'strawberry vagina' due to punctate hemorrhages. The cervix should be inspected for evidence of erosion, ectropion, ulcer, polyp or growth.

❖ A bimanual examination should always be performed to rule out uterine and adnexal pathology (such as PID).

❖ The discharge should be sent for microscopic examination and culture.

❖ Pap smear should be taken for cytology in the absence of obvious inflammation.

INVESTIGATIONS

❖ *Wet mount preparation*—To a drop of the discharge, a drop of saline is added and examined under the microscope. Motile, pear-shaped organisms are pathognomic of trichomonal infection. Presence of 'clue' cells (which are vaginal squamous cells showing stippling of cytoplasm due to adherent coccobacilli) points to gardnerella infection.

❖ *Potassium hydroxide (KOH) mount*—A drop of 10 per cent KOH is added to a drop of discharge and examined under the microscope. Presence of mycelia and spores suggests Candida albicans.

❖ *Whiff test*—Addition of KOH to vaginal secretion releases a fishy amine odour in gardnerella vaginitis.

❖ *Gram stain* of the discharge smeared on a slide can reveal Gram positive spores (in moniliasis) or Gram negative diplococci (in gonorrhea).

❖ *Culture of the discharge* for specific organisms may be needed. For trichomonas Stuart's medium, for Candida Nickerson's medium, and for gonococci Thayer–Martin medium are used.

❖ *Colposcopy* is useful in detecting premalignant lesions of the cervix, vagina and the vulva. Directed biopsies will confirm the nature of the lesion.

❖ Blood sugar estimation will help to exclude diabetes mellitus.

TREATMENT

 How should one proceed to treat this patient?

Measures should be instituted to improve the general condition of the patient, such as correction of anemia.

❖ Women with physiological discharge (especially unmarried girls) should be counselled and reassured.

❖ Improved genital hygiene should be emphasised.

❖ The male partner should be treated for genitourinary infection.

❖ For infection with trichomonas, *both partners should be treated* with metronidazole 200 mg TID for 7 days, or 400 mg BD for 5 days. When patient compliance seems uncertain, a single dose of 2 g of metronidazole may be used. However, it is likely to be less effective and may be repeated after a week.

❖ For moniliasis, a number of local and systemic medications are available, but the commonly used ones are clotrimazole (1%) cream 5 g intravaginally for 7–10 days or 100 mg vaginal tablets at bed time for 6 days. Fluconazole 150 mg single dose orally is very effective. In recurrent infections, the predisposing factors mentioned above (such as diabetes mellitus) should be carefully controlled.

❖ Bacterial vaginosis (Gardnerella vaginalis) is treated with metronidazole 400 mg BD for 7 days.

❖ Chlamydial infection is treated with doxycycline 100 mg BD for 10–14 days.

❖ Uncomplicated gonorrhea is treated with a single oral dose of norfloxacin 800 mg or ciprofloxacin 500 mg or cefixime 400 mg. Alternatively, a single injection of ceftriaxone 125 mg IM may be given.

❖ Senile vaginitis is treated with topical estrogen cream.

❖ Cervical erosion is treated by cryotherapy which may decrease glandular activity and thus decrease the discharge.

❖ Ectropion and chronic cervicitis sometimes require surgical treatment like trachelorrhaphy or partial amputation of cervix. Cervical polyps should be removed.

❖ Other lesions like neoplasia should be treated individually by specific therapy.

❖ If no definite cause is found for pruritus vulvae *general measures* like wearing cotton underclothing and antihistamines should be advised. Local application of hydrocortisone ointment alone or in combination with a fungicide, is helpful. If a specific skin condition is present, it should be treated.

Key points

1. Infection accounts for 90 per cent of cases presenting with white discharge. Trichomonas vaginalis and candida are the organisms frequently responsible for the infections.

2. Investigation and treatment of the male partner is essential.

3. Adequate attention should be paid to systemic disorders which adversely influence the outcome of specific therapy.

4. Pruritus vulvae is an additional symptom in patients with white discharge. In older women, pruritus vulvae could be a predominant symptom that requires to be investigated systematically.

5. Treatment is directed towards the cause. If no cause is found, therapeutic intervention is adopted to provide relief from symptoms.

CHAPTER 28

Irregular vaginal bleeding

S. HABEEBULLAH

S. SOUNDARA RAGHAVAN

In gynecological practice, one often encounters patients presenting with what they describe as 'irregular vaginal bleeding'. On detailed inquiry, most of these patients may have slight disturbances in the regularity of their menstrual cycles within the accepted limits of the normal menstrual cycle (21–35 days). Though the duration of menstrual cycles in a particular woman remains fairly constant, it may not be uncommon to find variations of a few days between menstrual cycles. What should be of concern is gross variation of cycle duration associated with increased blood loss, particularly, when it is severe enough to disturb the general condition. Prolongation of the cycle duration may also be important since it may indicate early stages of conditions causing amenorrhea. Shortening of the duration of menstrual cycles, if it occurs for long periods of time, may result in significant anemia even if the bleeding is within normal limits. However, *acyclical bleeding is a common presenting symptom of genital tract malignancies* and deserves thorough evaluation.

Objectives

At the end of this chapter, the reader should be able to

- ❏ Appreciate that irregular vaginal bleeding is a common problem.
- ❏ Enumerate the causes of irregular vaginal bleeding.
- ❏ Elicit appropriate history.
- ❏ Interpret findings of physical examination.
- ❏ Choose the investigations and interpret the results.
- ❏ Outline the management.

CLINICAL SCENARIO

A 28-year-old multiparous woman presents with a complaint of irregular vaginal bleeding of two years duration.

HISTORY

 ### What questions should be asked to gain a better understanding of the case?

The term irregular vaginal bleeding is used by patients to describe many types of menstrual abnormalities. Apart from including minor normal variations in the duration of menstrual cycles, they also include variations in the duration of menstrual bleeding.

❖ *Pattern of bleeding*—It is important to elicit a detailed menstrual history. It is often worthwhile to find out the exact dates of bleeding episodes if possible. It is surprising how poor the memory of patients is regarding their menstrual cycles. When the general condition of the patient is reasonable, it is useful to ask them to maintain a '*menstrual diary*' or '*menstrual calendar*' for three months, clearly indicating the '*bleeding free*' and '*bleeding*' days. This chart will help assign the pattern of bleeding to any of the following type:

Polymenorrhea (epimenorrhea)	:	Shortened cycles, normal bleeding
Oligomenorrhea	:	Prolonged cycles, normal bleeding
Menorrhagia	:	Normal cycles, prolonged or excess bleeding
Polymenorrhagia	:	Shortened cycles, prolonged or excess bleeding
Hypomenorrhea	:	Normal cycles, reduced bleeding days or reduced bleeding
Metrorrhagia	:	Loss of cyclicity or intermenstrual bleeding
Metropathia hemorrhagica	:	Periods of amenorrhea followed by prolonged bleeding, normal cycles followed by excess continuous bleeding, cycles with excess bleeding followed by continuous bleeding

❖ *Age*—The causes of irregular bleeding are usually different in different age groups.

In children and adolescents, irregular bleeding could be related to trauma by foreign bodies, sexual assault, use of exogenous hormones, bleeding disorders, anovulation and sometimes disturbed pregnancy. One may rarely encounter neoplasms like mixed mesodermal tumours of the vagina. In the *reproductive age group*, pregnancy related conditions, cervical lesions like erosion, cervical polyps, cancer of the uterine cervix and genital ulcers due to STDs are common. In the *postmenopausal age group*, cancer of the uterine cervix, cancer of endometrium, senile vaginitis, cancer of vagina, endometritis, decubitus ulcers and use of hormones should be kept in mind.

❖ *Parity*—Cancer cervix is more common in women with high parity, whereas fibroid polyp and endometrial cancer are common in those with low parity.

❖ *Postcoital bleeding*—It is important to inquire about episodes of postcoital bleeding; it could be due to a local lesion in the vagina or cervix, especially cervical carcinoma.

❖ *Menstrual history*—The amount of bleeding, duration of bleeding and interval between bleeding are noted. A history of amenorrhea may be present in PCOS, metropathia hemorrhagica and pregnancy related causes.

❖ *Contraceptive use*—Irregular use of OC pills or use of IUCD may be associated with irregular bleeding per vaginum. Progestogen-only contraceptive can also cause irregular bleeding.

❖ *Exogenous hormones*—History of irregular intake of estrogen or progestogen may also cause irregular bleeding.

❖ History of *sexually transmitted disease* or multiple sexual partners may indicate presence of lower genital tract lesions.

❖ Past or family history suggestive of *tuberculosis* may indicate tuberculous endometritis which can cause irregular bleeding. A history of diabetes mellitus and hypertension may be present in endometrial carcinoma.

PHYSICAL EXAMINATION

General examination—The presence of pallor may correlate with the severity of bleeding. Obesity and hirsutism are characteristics of polycystic ovarian syndrome. Thyromegaly should be noted. Lymphadenopathy may be present in tuberculosis or malignancies.

Abdominal examination—This may reveal a mass.

Speculum examination—A careful speculum examination should be performed to look for lesions on the cervix, like erosion, which has a velvety appearance. Cancer may present as a proliferative growth or an ulcer on the cervix or the vagina. A polyp may be seen protruding from the cervical os. The appearance of the vagina in trichomonal infection is described as punctate vaginitis, due to minute hemorrhages (strawberry appearance in severe infection).

Bimanual vaginal examination—This may reveal an enlarged uterus due to a fibroid or cancer endometrium. The size of the uterus is unchanged in senile endometritis. There is blood on the examining finger in case of a lesion on the cervix and the vagina. A soft enlarged uterus suggests pregnancy associated conditions. The fornices should be thoroughly palpated to check for adnexal mass or bogginess suggestive of ectopic gestation.

Rectal examination—This is performed with the aim of detecting infiltration of the parametrium or uterosacral ligaments in case of cervical or vaginal and ovarian cancer.

INVESTIGATIONS

❖ Complete hemogram including peripheral smear.

❖ Pap smear is useful in detecting premalignant or malignant lesions of the cervix which are not clinically obvious. If the smear is positive, a directed biopsy using colposcopy or Schiller's test is indicated. In some women, particularly postmenopausal, a cone biopsy needs to be performed.

❖ If a growth is present, it should be biopsied.

❖ Ultrasonography, preferably transvaginal, will confirm the presence of submucous fibroid and polycystic ovaries. Endometrial thickness can be assessed in order to plan further investigations for confirmation of endometrial cancer.

❖ Fractional curettage is useful for diagnosing endometrial and endocervical cancer.

❖ Hysteroscopy will confirm submucous fibroid and endometrial cancer.

❖ Estimation of serum LH and FSH is useful if PCOS is suspected; the ratio of LH:FSH will be 3:1 or more.

❖ Thyroid function tests are indicated if there is clinical suspicion of thyroid dysfunction.

❖ Urine for pregnancy test or serum estimation of β hCG is called for when ectopic pregnancy is suspected.

TREATMENT

 How should one proceed to treat this patient?

❖ The general condition should be improved and specific treatment directed towards the cause.

❖ In the adolescent age group, after excluding pregnancy and local conditions, the treatment consists of cyclical progestogens assuming the cause to be anovulatory bleeding. If contraception is needed, oral pills are advised. Abortions should be treated as indicated (see Chapter 6).

❖ Cervical erosion, after exclusion of malignancy, can be treated with cryocautery. Premalignant lesions of the cervix may be treated with ablative or excisional procedures or hysterectomy.

❖ Cancer cervix is probably the commonest cause of irregular vaginal bleeding due to malignancy among women of reproductive or menopausal age group. Its treatment should be planned with the radiotherapist, as the option of surgery or radiotherapy depends on factors like clinical stage of disease, pathological type of tumour and age.

❖ Malignancies of various sites are managed according to specific protocols.

❖ If no pathology is detected, these patients can be reassured. The variations that can occur in the normal menstrual cycles and the possibility of ovulation spotting should be explained.

They should also be assured that they will be followed up, examined at regular intervals, and investigated if necessary to exclude abnormalities.

It is useful to suggest to all girls and women of reproductive age group to maintain a menstrual diary or a calendar. At each visit, this diary can be used to ascertain the type of bleeding. This is a simple and useful tool to help keep track of menstrual problems.

Key points

1. Irregular bleeding per vaginum may be caused by lesions ranging from an erosion to a cervical cancer.
2. History of postcoital bleeding must always be enquired into.
3. A vaginal speculum examination is useful in determining the cause of irregular bleeding.

4. It is mandatory to take a Pap smear for all sexually active women.
5. In women of reproductive age, disturbed pregnancy, use of IUCDs and progestogen contraceptives are common causes of irregular bleeding per vaginum.
6. The commonest cause of postmenopausal bleeding in India continues to be cervical cancer.

CHAPTER 29

Excessive vaginal bleeding

S. HABEEBULLAH

The average amount of blood loss during normal menstruation is about 80 ml. Menorrhagia is excessive menstrual bleeding, either in quantity or in duration (more than seven days) without alteration in the length of the cycle. It is a common presenting symptom and a cause for anemia in women of the reproductive age group. The most common cause of menorrhagia is dysfunctional uterine bleeding (DUB).

Objectives

At the end of this chapter, the reader should be able to

- ❑ Enumerate the causes of menorrhagia in different age groups.
- ❑ Define DUB.
- ❑ Elicit appropriate history and perform physical examination.
- ❑ List the investigations to establish the diagnosis.
- ❑ Outline the management.

CLINICAL SCENARIO

A 32-year-old woman, presents with complaints of excessive bleeding per vaginum.

 Could this patient be suffering from DUB?

Dysfunctional uterine bleeding is diagnosed if no organic cause is detected; there is no palpable pelvic pathology. The diagnosis is by exclusion. Pregnancy associated conditions, tumours and inflammatory conditions should be excluded by clinical methods or investigations.

DUB can be classified as ovular and anovular types:

1. Ovular type
    Functional epimenorrhea or epimenorrhagia
    Corpus luteum abnormalities:
        Irregular ripening
        Irregular shedding
2. Anovular type
    Metropathia hemorrhagica

HISTORY

 What questions should be asked to gain a better understanding of the case?

Whenever a woman presents with excessive bleeding per vaginum, a thorough history is very useful.

* ❖ *Age*—This patient is in the reproductive age group when fibroids, endometriosis and pelvic inflammatory disease (PID) occur more frequently. Dysfunctional uterine bleeding (DUB) is more common at the extremes of reproductive life. In perimenopausal patients, in addition to the above conditions, the possibility of endometrial carcinoma should be kept in mind.
* ❖ *Drugs*—Whenever a woman presents with excessive or irregular bleeding, one must enquire about ingestion of hormones, especially estrogens.
* ❖ *Parity*—Fibroid uterus and endometriosis are more common in nulliparous women. Patients suffering from adenomyosis are usually parous.
* ❖ One must routinely ask about IUCD insertion; excessive bleeding occurs in some women using these devices.
* ❖ *Menstrual history* must be taken very carefully; it should include information about the length of menstrual cycles, and duration and amount of blood flow. The length of the cycles is increased in case of metropathia hemorrhagica; the woman complains of 2–3 months of amenorrhea followed by excessive bleeding. Normal length of cycle and excessive bleeding suggest fibroid uterus, endometriosis and PID.

The presence of clots in the menstrual discharge confirms that the woman is actually suffering from menorrhagia. One could confirm this by enquiring about the number of vulval pads/vaginal tampons used.

❖ *Dysmenorrhea* can be of two types—congestive and spasmodic. The congestive type, starts before the onset of menstruation and is relieved once the menstruation starts. It is characteristically associated with endometriosis and PID. The spasmodic type is experienced particularly by women suffering from a submucous fibroid, and also by those using an IUCD. Anovular DUB is painless.

❖ *Dyspareunia* is frequently associated with endometriosis and PID.

❖ It is essential to elicit symptoms suggestive of hypothyroidism, bleeding diathesis and tuberculosis. Menorrhagia is present in the initial phase of endometrial tuberculosis in 10 per cent of cases.

PHYSICAL EXAMINATION

Obesity, anemia, thyroid swelling, and hypertension should be looked for. Abdominal examination may reveal hepatosplenomegaly or masses arising from the pelvis, like fibroid uterus. On pelvic examination, the uterus is either of normal size or enlarged uniformly up to eight weeks' size, and is non-tender in case of DUB. In adenomyosis, the uterus is tender and uniformly enlarged, but not larger than 10–12 weeks' size. In the presence of a fibroid, the uterus is usually irregularly enlarged. In women suffering from PID and endometriosis, the uterus may be of normal size, and tender, with restricted mobility; adnexal masses may be palpable and tender. Rectal examination also confirms tenderness of uterosacral ligaments due to endometriotic deposits.

INVESTIGATIONS

Investigations should be directed towards finding a cause in the genital tract and generalised disease for menorrhagia, to enable rational treatment.

❖ Complete hemogram including peripheral smear, bleeding time and clotting time should be done. This will help in determining the type and severity of anemia and also to rule out the possibility of bleeding diathesis.

❖ Thyroid function tests (TSH, T_3 and T_4) will rule out hypothyroidism or thyrotoxicosis.

❖ Ultrasonography helps assess the size of the uterus, and detect any tumours or bicornuate uterus and adnexal mass. Adenomyosis can be suspected using (preferably) transvaginal sonography. Endometrial thickness should be measured.

If it is found to be abnormally thickened, especially in a perimenopausal woman, one must consider the possibility of endometrial cancer and plan further investigation.

❖ Fractional curettage will not only rule out malignancy but will also indicate the histological pattern of the endometrium—proliferative, secretory or hyperplastic with or without atypia.

❖ For diagnosis of irregular ripening, dilatation and curettage (D and C) should be done premenstrually or on the first day of menstruation when the endometrium shows patchy secretory changes. In case of irregular shedding, the endometrium shows persistent secretory changes along with proliferation, on day five or six.

❖ Hysteroscopy can detect small submucous fibroid, endometrial polyp and malignancy.

❖ Therapeutic D and C is indicated in a patient who is bleeding profusely. Curettage removes most of the functional layer of endometrium and controls the bleeding in that particular cycle. **It is mandatory to send the curettings for histopathological examination.**

TREATMENT

 How should one proceed to treat this patient?

❖ *General measures* include treatment of anemia, if present, by hematinics and in severe cases, by blood transfusion.

❖ *Fibroid uterus*—In younger patients and those desirous of bearing a child, myomectomy is advised. Hysterectomy should be considered in older women.

❖ *PID* can be treated with antibiotics (example, doxycycline) and NSAIDs. If symptoms persist with non-resolving adnexal masses, they should be surgically removed.

❖ *Endometriosis* can be treated with drugs like danazol (200–600 mg/day) for six months, or progestogens, used when necessary in combination with surgery to remove endometriotic lesions like chocolate cysts. In perimenopausal patients' total abdominal hysterectomy with bilateral salpingo-oophorectomy is the surgery of choice.

❖ *Adenomyosis* usually does not respond to hormones and hysterectomy is the only measure to provide relief.

✤ Anovulatory bleeding is the most common and if the patient is also infertile, ovulation induction using clomiphene citrate is the treatment of choice. In others progestogens like medroxy progesterone acetate 10 mg is prescribed daily from day 16–25 for 3–6 cycles.

Ovulatory bleeding can be treated by using combined OC pills for 3–6 cycles, or by mefenamic acid (500 mg TID) during menstruation, or by antifibrinolytic agents like tranexamic acid. Irregular ripening can be treated by progestogens in the second half of the menstrual cycle.

When the patient presents with acute bleeding, medroxy progesterone (30–40 mg per day) is used till bleeding stops. The dose is reduced to 10–20 mg/day for 10–14 days. After that, progestogens can be used cyclically from day 16–25 as described above.

Though patients with atypical hyperplasia of the endometrium can be treated with high-dose progestogens, hysterectomy should be the treatment of choice in view of the 25–30 per cent risk of endometrial cancer, particularly in the perimenopausal age group.

ROLE OF SURGERY IN DUB

Perimenopausal patients not responding to medical therapy, or those with poor compliance are candidates for hysterectomy. Wherever possible, vaginal hysterectomy should be performed.

Currently, alternative modalities like transcervical endometrial resection (TCER) and endometrial ablation using laser or radiofrequency endometrial ablation are also available. These procedures carry a failure rate of about 10 per cent depending on the experience of the surgeon.

Key points

1. Excessive bleeding per vaginum is a debilitating symptom.
2. A careful elicitation of history and thorough clinical examination help to detect the underlying cause.
3. Investigations are useful for general evaluation of the patient and to detect the cause of excessive bleeding.
4. A diagnosis of DUB should be made only after excluding an organic cause.
5. Medical management is preferred in younger patients; if surgery is required, a conservative method should be selected.
6. Hysterectomy is a plausible option in perimenopausal women.

CHAPTER 30

Absence of menstruation

GITA RAJAGOPALAN

Amenorrhea, or absence of menstruation is a condition that causes anxiety. If menstruation never started at all, it is termed *primary amenorrhea*. If there has been cessation of menses after a period of regular menstruation, it is called *secondary amenorrhea*. While amenorrhea may be caused by simple physiological states like pregnancy or lactation, serious conditions like ovarian tumours and intracranial lesions may also present as amenorrhea. Sometimes it is possible to identify the cause easily, but in other situations, elaborate and extensive investigations may be needed.

Objectives

At the end of this chapter, the reader should be able to

- ❑ Define primary and secondary amenorrhea.
- ❑ Elicit relevant history in a patient with amenorrhea.
- ❑ Perform appropriate clinical examination.
- ❑ Choose relevant investigations systematically.
- ❑ Plan treatment for amenorrhea.

CLINICAL SCENARIO

A 16-year-old girl presents with the complaint of not having attained menarche. She appears very short and has a pigeon chest.

Could this girl be suffering from primary amenorrhea?

Since the girl is sixteen years old and she has failed to attain menarche, she may be classified as having primary amenorrhea. Primary amenorrhea can be diagnosed in even a 14-year-old girl if she has absolutely no development of secondary sex characteristics like breasts, axillary and pubic hair and development of external genitalia.

 When is secondary amenorrhea diagnosed?

If there is a definite history of menstruation occurring earlier and there has been cessation of menstruation for a period of six months or a period equal to the duration of three menstrual cycles, secondary amenorrhea is diagnosed.

HISTORY

 What questions must be asked to gain a better understanding of the case?

First of all, it is essential to establish that menstruation has truly occurred for a while, particularly in young girls. Often, occasional episodes of staining or spotting are reported as menstruation.

* ♣ The patient may be asked if she suffers from any *abdominal pain*. To begin with, there may be regular cyclical monthly lower abdominal pain followed by almost continuous pain. Sometimes there may be retention of urine. These may suggest that there is 'hidden menstruation' or 'cryptomenorrhea'. In such a case, due to some obstruction in the outflow tract, menstrual blood accumulates in the vagina or the uterus, causing a *pelvic swelling* like hematocolpos or hematometra.

* ♣ Further, enquiry should be made regarding history of *headaches, visual disturbances* or *secretion from the breasts*. These indicate the presence of an intracranial lesion like pituitary adenoma. History of intolerance to cold, constipation and lethargy suggest hypothyroidism.

* ♣ Features of *defeminisation* or *virilisation* like voice change, abnormal hair distribution or growth, and enlargement of clitoris should be enquired into. They are present in congenital adrenal hyperplasia.

* ♣ Since many causes of primary amenorrhea may be developmental or due to chromosomal defects, *similar history in the family* or history of infertility in female

siblings is relevant. The chromosomal characteristics causing amenorrhea are given below.

A. Chromosomally competent

I.   *46 XX*   a) Eugonadotrophic

                    1. Normal stature

                        Outflow tract abnormalities

                        Mullerian agenesis

                        Asherman syndrome

                        Imperforate hymen

                        Sequelae of meningitis or encephalitis

                    2. Short stature

                        Pituitary dwarfism

                        Lorain–Levi syndrome

                        Lawrence–Moon–Biedl syndrome

                b) Hypergonadotrophic

                        Pituitary micro or macroadenomas

                c) Hypogonadotrophic

                        Physiological – delayed puberty

                        Hypothalamopituitary dysfunction

                        Kallman syndrome (GnRH)

II.   *46 XY*   Androgen insensitivity syndrome (testicular feminisation)

B. Chromosomally incompetent

46 XO and mosaics   Turner syndrome and variants

❖ An attempt should also be made to explore whether the girl is under any psychological stress. Excess physical activity such as in athletes can also delay menarche.

❖ It is very important to probe carefully and elicit history to exclude pregnancy and associated conditions. Pregnancy is the commonest cause of secondary amenorrhea in the reproductive age. Sometimes the patient may attempt to conceal such information. Intense desire to become pregnant may cause amenorrhea and other pregnancy symptoms in a condition called *pseudocyesis*.

❖ History of repeated induced abortions and D and C may lead to destruction of the endometrium, causing amenorrhea. The age of the last child, and whether the woman is lactating should be found out to exclude lactational amenorrhea.

❖ History of postpartum hemorrhage and failure of lactation in the preceding pregnancy may point to *Sheehan syndrome* due to anterior pituitary failure.

❖ History of loss of weight and appetite, fever and night sweats and contact with tuberculosis will help to diagnose tuberculosis, which is widely prevalent in India.

❖ Weight gain, pimples, slightly excess hair growth and pigmentation of skin may suggest polycystic ovarian syndrome (PCOS).

❖ Anorexia nervosa is a condition when there is a compulsive desire to starve and fasting is obsessional. It is usually seen in young adolescents.

❖ Enquiry should be made regarding vaginal dryness, dyspareunia, hot flushes and mood swings which may indicate premature menopause.

The causes of secondary amenorrhea are briefly listed below:

1. Central nervous system
   ✦ Psychogenic causes – anorexia nervosa, stress, anxiety states, pseudocyesis
   ✦ Infections – encephalitis, meningitis
   ✦ Drugs – reserpine, methyldopa, cimetedine, haloperidol and phenothiazines; injectable/implant progestins, combined oral contaceptive pills (postpill amenorrhea) and centchroman
   ✦ Pituitary tumours – prolactinomas, adenomas
   ✦ Pituitary necrosis – Simmonds disease, Sheehan syndrome

2. Ovary
   ✦ Premature ovarian failure
   ✦ Polycystic ovarian syndrome
   ✦ Virilising ovarian tumours – arrhenoblastoma, hilus cell tumours

3. Uterus
   ✦ Asherman syndrome
   ✦ Tuberculous endometritis

4. Other causes
   ✦ Thyroid and adrenal dysfunction
   ✦ Chronic liver and kidney diseases

EXAMINATION

The patient's height, weight, armspan, development of breasts, axillary and pubic hair and external genitalia are noted.

Pigeon chest, webbing of neck, cubitus valgus and coarctation of aorta suggest Turner syndrome. Presence of galactorrhea may indicate hypothyroidism or hyper-prolactinemia. A lower abdominal mass may be due to hematometra.

Gynecological examination

Non-development of external genitalia suggests hypogonadism. Clitoral enlargement and presence of inguinal hernias will favour testicular feminisation syndrome.

If the hymen can be seen bulging, shining and bluish, the diagnosis is imperforate hymen.

In a woman who has been previously normal, atrophy of the vulva, loss of rugosity, and dryness of the vagina before the age of 40 years will suggest premature menopause.

A proper vaginal examination, where possible, will help to identify an early pregnancy, atrophic uterus or an ovarian tumour. If vaginal examination is not possible, rectal examination should be performed to palpate the cervix, uterus or any other mass.

INVESTIGATIONS

❖ Ultrasonography helps to confirm pregnancy and mullerian duct agenesis.

❖ Karyotyping is an essential test for suspected Turner syndrome, testicular feminisation syndrome, or those with mullerian duct failure.

❖ CT scan or MRI of the skull will be useful in diagnosing intracranial lessions.

❖ Hormone estimations should be specifically chosen to diagnose conditions like PCOS, adrenal hyperplasia and premature ovarian failure. FSH levels are raised in premature ovarian failure and LH:FSH ratio is 3:1 or more in PCOS when estimated on day 2 or day 3 of menstrual cycle.

❖ Fasting levels of blood glucose and insulin will help to identify hyperinsulinemia.

❖ Thyroid functions will help to diagnose thyroid abnormalities. Prolactin levels are raised in case of prolactinomas.

❖ Estimation of b hCG and/or ultrasonography will help to exclude pregnancy and related conditions in case of secondary amenorrhea.

❖ Chest x-ray is useful in detecting pulmonary tuberculosis.

❖ Endometrial biopsy must be taken and sent for histological examination and culture to confirm or rule out genital tuberculosis.

❖ Diagnostic laparoscopy is useful for evaluation of the tubes and ovaries. Presence of tubercles suggests genital tuberculosis.

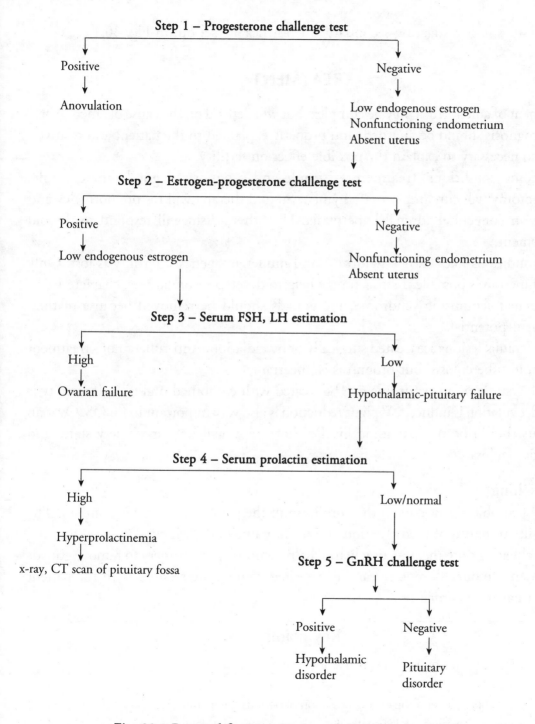

Fig. 30.1 Protocol for investigation of secondary amenorrhea

The steps in investigating secondary amenorrhea are set out in Fig. 30.1.

TREATMENT

Treatment of amenorrhea may be complex, but will depend on the cause of amenorrhea. The prognosis should be guarded, and properly explained to the patient and relatives. It is also necessary to explain the possible effect on fertility.

In some conditions, treatment is simple and prognosis is good. For example, hymenotomy will cure imperforate hymen. Steroid therapy will restore normalcy and fertility in congenital adrenal hyperplasia. Hypothyroidism will respond to thyroid replacement.

In conditions like Turner syndrome and mullerian agenesis, fertility is lost. Only coital function is possible. Estrogen may help to develop secondary sex characteristics. In testicular feminising syndrome, the gonads should be removed because of their malignant potential.

Intracranial lesions are treated surgically or by radiation. Anti-tuberculous treatment is given in tuberculosis, but prognosis is uncertain.

Polycystic ovarian syndrome can be treated with combined oral pills. If fertility is desired, ovulation is induced. Weight reduction is also very important in PCOS. Ovarian tumours should be treated surgically. Psychotherapy will help in anxiety states and anorexia nervosa.

Counselling

It is best to objectively explain the condition to the patient and/or the guardian. The possibility of return of menstruation and fertility must be clarified. The need for long term or lifelong drug therapy, psychiatric help, neurosurgery, surgery to remove gonads or ovarian tumours all require careful, repeated counselling sessions with the patient and her partner/guardian.

Key points

1. Primary amenorrhea is defined as the failure to attain menarche by 16 years of age.
2. Secondary amenorrhea is the cessation of periods for six months.
3. Primary amenorrhea is usually due to a developmental defect.

4. Cryptomenorrhea is usually due to imperforate hymen.
5. Consider the possibility of pregnancy in secondary amenorrhea.
6. There is a significant prevalence of genital tuberculosis in India.
7. Cases of amenorrhea need to be investigated and managed systematically.
8. Loss of menstruation and fertility causes considerable anxiety and requires proper counselling.

CHAPTER 31

Mass descending per vaginum

P. REDDI RANI

Mass descending per vaginum is a common gynecological complaint and is often due to uterovaginal prolapse. It results from defective pelvic supports allowing the vagina, uterus and adjacent organs to descend below their normal anatomical position. It is seen frequently in women in the peri/postmenopausal age group and is attributed to declining levels of estrogens. Uterovaginal prolapse is occasionally seen in young girls or women and is associated with spina bifida or congenital weakness of pelvic floor muscles and ligaments.

Objectives

At the end of this chapter, the reader should be able to

❑ Define the various types of vaginal prolapse and uterine descent.

❑ Explain the cause of uterovaginal prolapse.

❑ Enumerate the common symptoms.

❑ Differentiate uterovaginal prolapse from other causes of mass descending per vaginum.

❑ Appreciate that preventive measures can be effective.

❑ Select appropriate investigations.

❑ Suggest management options in different age groups.

CLINICAL SCENARIO

A 45-year-old multiparous woman presents with mass descending per vaginum of one year duration, with difficulty in passing urine.

HISTORY

 What questions must be asked to gain a better understanding of the case?

In a perimenopausal woman, the common activating factors in the presence of birth injury and postmenopausal tissue atrophy are chronic cough, constipation, ascites and large abdominal tumours. A detailed obstetric history, with particular attention to factors like pregnancies at short intervals, unattended deliveries, operative vaginal deliveries and birth of big babies, prolonged second stage and lack of perineal exercises in the postnatal period should be elicited.

The connective tissue that is compressed to form fascial support to the vagina, bladder or rectum may be weakened when there is malnutrition or deficiency of estrogen around the time of menopause. When connective tissue fails, muscular support will be weak, leading to widening of the urogenital hiatus in the pelvic diaphragm. This predisposes to descent of the uterus and vagina. Of particular importance is the tone of the puborectalis muscle (Fig. 31.1).

❖ History of urinary problems like difficulty in initiating micturition, is common. With a large cystocele, it is difficult to empty the bladder; the more the patient strains the greater the difficulty, as the bladder base and the trigone descend below the level of the urethra. She can empty the bladder only after reducing the mass digitally. Incomplete emptying of the bladder leads to increase in frequency and to dysuria due to cystitis. Rarely, the patient could present with retention of urine. Stress urinary incontinence could also be one of the complaints.

❖ Difficulty in emptying the rectum suggests the presence of rectocele.

❖ Presence of leucorrhea, metrorrhagia, or postcoital bleeding point to decubitus ulcer which is usually benign; it is present on the dependent portion, and is caused by tissue anoxia due to venous stasis.

❖ Irreducibility of the mass is often due to congestion, edema and hypertrophy of tissues in longstanding cases.

❖ It is important to elicit menstrual history in detail as it will indicate any need for investigations, and also governs the choice of treatment.

❖ Parity of the patient, and the desire to preserve reproductive and menstrual function should be enquired into, as the choice of type of surgery depends on all these factors.

❖ History of chronic cough is important; if present, the cough should be treated prior to surgery.

❖ Past history of wearing a pessary, or any attempts at repair of the prolapse are important in planning the treatment.

PHYSICAL EXAMINATION

General examination

The general condition of the patient should be assessed. The respiratory system must be checked to rule out any chronic respiratory illness which presents as chronic cough.

Abdominal examination

This should include a careful inspection of hernial sites and palpation to detect any mass.

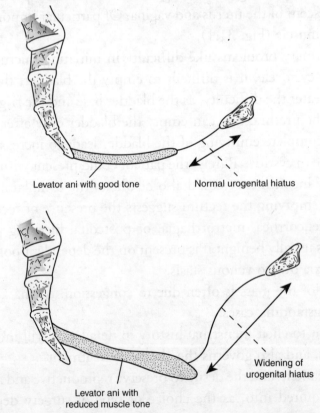

Levator ani with good tone   Normal urogenital hiatus

Widening of urogenital hiatus

Levator ani with reduced muscle tone

Fig. 31.1 Role of muscle tone in the causation of uterovaginal prolapse

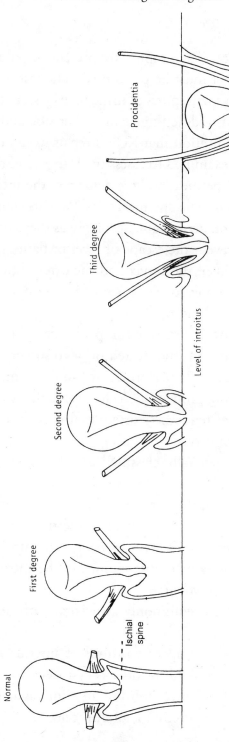
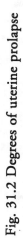

Normal

First degree

Ischial spine

Level of introitus

Second degree

Third degree

Procidentia

Fig. 31.2 Degrees of uterine prolapse

Pelvic examination

❖ Stress urinary incontinence, if symptoms are present, should be elicited with full bladder and a Bonney's test must be performed. The test is performed by asking the woman to strain when small spurts of urine may be seen; then the bladder neck is elevated with index and middle fingers on either side and if the spurt of urine does not occur, it is an indication that Kelly's repair would be effective.

❖ The perineum should be examined to assess the integrity of the perineal body and tone of the levator ani. If perineal body is damaged, the introitus will be lax and there may be evidence of old healed perineal tears. Patients with third degree perineal tears are unlikely to develop uterovaginal prolapse as they constantly exercise their pelvic floor muscles to prevent the escape of feces or flatus.

❖ Note the degree of descent of the cervix and the extent of cystocele, urethrocele, enterocele and rectocele. Look for evidence of hypertrophy, congestion, edema, decubitus ulcer and keratinisation.

Vaginal mucosa must be inspected for presence of infection or atrophy. If present, these conditions must be treated prior to surgery.

Bimanual pelvic examination is performed to note the direction of the uterus. A retroverted uterus is more prone to descent. Note the size and mobility of the uterus and the presence of tenderness or adnexal mass in the fornices, as well as supravaginal elongation of cervix.

❖ Uterovaginal prolapse is generally classified as follows (Fig. 31.2). The normal position of cervix is at the level of ischial spines.

First degree—The descent of the cervix is below the level of ischial spines.

Second degree—The descent of the cervix is up to the introitus.

Third degree—The descent of the cervix is below the introitus.

Fourth degree—The fundus of uterus is outside the introitus. This degree of descent is also known as *procidentia*.

Prolapse of the vaginal wall is commonly associated with descent of the adjacent organs (Fig. 31.3):

Anterior vaginal wall   –   upper two-thirds of anterior vaginal wall with bladder is cystocele

–   lower third of anterior vaginal wall with urethra is urethrocele

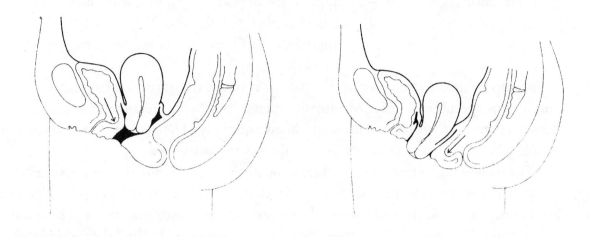

Fig. 31.3 a: Cystocele   Fig. 31.3 b: Rectocele

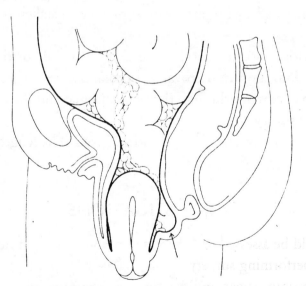

Fig. 31.3 c: Enterocele

Reproduced with permission from *Illustrated Textbook of Gynaecology.*
Mackay EV, Beischer NA,
Pepperell RJ and Wood C (Eds.) 2nd ed, WB Saunders and Bailliere Tindall, 1992, p 347.

Posterior vaginal wall –   upper third of post vaginal wall with intestines
is enterocele
middle third of post vaginal wall with rectum is
rectocele

In order to detect an enterocele, the patient is put in the dorsal/left lateral position, and a Sims speculum is inserted into the vagina so as to depress the rectocele. The cervix is then held with a vulsellum and lifted anteriorly. The patient is now asked to cough; a bulge beyond the tip of the speculum is the enterocele.

❖ The patient under discussion is likely to be suffering from third degree uterovaginal prolapse or procidentia, since there is a large cystocele as she has difficulty in passing urine. If the thumb and the fingers can be approximated at the introitus (getting above the swelling), the patient has a procidentia. In third degree prolapse, it is not possible to get above the swelling.

DIFFERENTIAL DIAGNOSIS

Other conditions to be differentiated from uterovaginal prolapse are:

❖ Anterior vaginal wall cyst (Gartner cyst) may be mistaken for a cystocele but it is not reducible.

❖ Congenital elongation of cervix where the vaginal fornices are deep, unlike supravaginal elongation in uterovaginal prolapse.

❖ Fibroid polyp comes out through the cervical canal and the cervical lips can be felt all around the pedicle.

❖ Chronic inversion is usually due to fundal fibroid. The length of the uterine cavity is shortened.

INVESTIGATIONS

❖ Anemia should be assessed and corrected preoperatively if necessary as there is no urgency for performing surgery.

❖ Urine for albumin, sugar and microscopic examination are indicated to detect diabetes, urinary tract infection and renal disorders.

❖ Urine for culture and sensitivity should be done if the patient is symptomatic, or if microscopy reveals pus cells.

❖ Urinary tract infection if present should be treated preoperatively, to avoid the exacerbation of infection which occurs postoperatively, especially since the patient will be on continuous bladder drainage for 24–48 hours.

❖ Other investigations like blood urea and creatinine, X-ray chest and ECG should be carried out in patients of the older age group, as a part of surgical work up.

❖ Pap smear should ideally be done in all the cases especially in those above 35 years of age and those with decubitus ulcers. Biopsy of the cervix for non-healing ulcers and that of the endometrium for abnormal bleeding should be done.

❖ Intravenous pyelogram is indicated only in longstanding cases of irreducible procidentia. Even if hydronephrosis and hydroureter are present, they usually return to normal once the uterovaginal prolapse is treated.

TREATMENT

 How does one proceed to treat this patient?

Pre-operative preparation

Correction of anemia and treatment of urinary tract infection are absolutely essential. Decubital ulcer is treated by reducing the prolapse and plugging the vagina with tampon soaked in acriflavine and glycerine. This reduces the tissue edema, restores circulation, and helps the healing of a decubitus ulcer. If a woman is postmenopausal and tissues are atrophic, local estrogen cream for 2–3 weeks is useful in increasing the thickness of vagina.

Surgical management

Treatment depends on several factors like age, parity, type of prolapse, desire to preserve reproductive and menstrual function and presence of any associated pathology. The objective is surgical restoration of normal anatomy.

Anterior colporrhaphy is performed for prolapse of the anterior vaginal wall. It is combined with Kelly's repair if there is associated stress incontinence.

For patients below 40 years of age who desire preservation of reproductive and menstrual function, the treatment of choice is **Manchester operation** which consists of (a) partial amputation of the cervix, (b) shortening of the Mackenrodt's ligaments and resuturing these ligaments in front of the cervix to make the uterus anteverted, combined with (c) anterior colporrhaphy and (d) colpoperineorrhaphy. If the patient desires permanent contraception, tubectomy can be performed either vaginally or abdominally. In the older age group or in those with other pelvic pathology, vaginal hysterectomy with pelvic floor repair (Ward–Mayo's operation) is the treatment of choice. If an enterocele is present, special care should be taken to repair it when performing Manchester or Ward–Mayo's operation.

Possible complications of surgery are:

❖ Hemorrhage and injury to the bladder and rectum may occur during surgery. Reactionary hemorrhage is not an uncommon complication in the first 24 hours. It is due to slippage of ligatures after the blood pressure is restored. The patient needs to be explored under anesthesia to secure hemostasis. In the postoperative period, urinary infection is common due to catheterisation and also if a preoperative infection was not treated. Other complications are vault infection and thrombophlebitis. Secondary hemorrhage is another important problem, which occurs 7–10 days postoperatively and is usually due to infection. Antibiotics and vaginal packing are usually effective.

❖ Late complications include recurrence of prolapse and vault prolapse; these may be attributed to an ill chosen operation and poor surgical technique, and omission to recognise and treat an enterocele. The other problem the patient can present with is dyspareunia due to early resumption of coitus before healing of tissues, too much narrowing of introitus or too short a vagina.

❖ Following Manchester operation there may be infertility, abortion and preterm labour due to cervical incompetence.

Role of pessary

This is indicated only during pregnancy, in puerperium or when the patient is not fit for surgery due to old age and/or medical complications. No young woman should ever be advised a pessary except in pregnancy. Wearing a pessary may cause more discomfort than having prolapse; it does not control stress incontinence and may cause ulceration of the vagina.

PREVENTION

Adequate spacing between pregnancies, limiting the number of children, avoidance of premature straining in first stage of labour, avoiding prolonged labour, adequate episiotomy when needed, proper repair of perineal and vaginal lacerations, early ambulation and avoiding excess physical strain in the puerperium may help in reducing the incidence of uterovaginal prolapse.

Connective tissue is composed of elastin and collagen fibres in polysaccharide ground substance. It forms capsules to maintain the structural integrity of the organs, including the muscles and the tendons. If connective tissue fails, muscular support will be weak. Hormonal changes during pregnancy, labour and menopause have significant effect on collagen. Exercise, and nutrition, particularly intake of vitamin C, are responsible for maintenance of connective tissue integrity.

Key points

1. Uterovaginal prolapse is a common gynecological condition.
2. Loss of tone of supporting tissue and ligaments, either congenital or due to childbirth and decline in estrogens around menopause lead to uterovaginal prolapse.
3. Urinary complications are frequent.
4. Treatment is essentially surgical, aimed at correcting the anatomical displacement.
5. Precautions during labour, exercise, and good nutrition are known to help in the prevention of uterovaginal prolapse.

CHAPTER 32

Mass lower abdomen

Asha Oumachigui

The causes of a lower abdominal mass are vastly different in the prepubertal period, during adolescence, the reproductive age group, or in the postmenopausal period. The mass may originate from the reproductive organs or it may arise from other structures like the urinary bladder or lymph nodes. A thorough history and physical examination, followed by appropriate laboratory investigations is critical in the management of lower abdominal mass.

Objectives

At the end of this chapter, the reader should be able to

- ❑ Take relevant history.
- ❑ Identify on general examination, features of certain typical conditions.
- ❑ Differentiate lower abdominal masses arising from different anatomical structures on abdominal, pelvic and rectal examination.
- ❑ Choose appropriate investigations to confirm the diagnosis or to detect any complications.

CLINICAL SCENARIO

A 35-year-old woman presents with the complaint of a mass in the lower abdomen.

HISTORY

✋ ***What questions should be asked to gain a better understanding of the case?***

❖ The age of the patient under discussion is 35 years; in this age group a fibroid uterus is common. Ovarian tumours if present would be benign in all probability. Below nine years of age and after menopause, the majority of ovarian tumours are likely to be malignant. In a young girl presenting with the symptom triad of amenorrhea, pain and mass abdomen the diagnosis is almost certainly hematometra. Further, age would be an important determinant of the treatment option. In case of the young or in those desirous of retaining reproductive or menstrual function, a conservative approach may be followed.

❖ The patient must be asked about the duration for which the mass has been present. Benign tumours like fibroids are likely to be present for a long time, sometimes for years. Rapid growth is indicative of malignant ovarian tumours; fibroid associated with pregnancy often grows rapidly.

❖ Excessive bleeding during periods and small intermenstrual bleeds are characteristic of fibroid uterus. Menorrhagia is due to an increase in endometrial surface and to some extent, endometrial hyperplasia due to hyperestrogenism. A submucous fibroid may present as intermenstrual bleeding caused by ulceration of the surface.

Abnormal uterine bleeding could be a presenting symptom of estrogen-producing ovarian tumours like the granulosa cell tumour. In a prepubertal girl, the parents may bring the child suspecting precocious puberty. In the reproductive age group, the pattern of bleeding resembles metropathia hemorrhagica and in elderly women, it may be postmenopausal bleeding.

Irregular bleeding associated with purulent discharge is characteristic of pyometra complicating cancer of the uterine cervix.

It is important to enquire about the date of the last menstrual period (LMP). If there is history of missed periods, one should suspect or rule out pregnancy in a woman of reproductive age.

❖ Pain is not always associated with a lower abdominal mass. However dysmenorrhea, both spasmodic and congestive is usually present in case of fibroid uterus. Dull aching pain could be due to large ovarian tumours, fibroids and inflammatory tubo-ovarian masses. Acute pain characterises complications of ovarian tumours such as torsion, infection, or hemorrhage and red degeneration of fibroids.

✤ Dyspepsia, characteristic of gastrointestinal disorders, is often the only symptom in patients with ovarian cancer. Many of these women consult a physician or general surgeon and are treated symptomatically.

A 65-year-old woman consulted a physician for dyspepsia; she was diagnosed to have gastritis and was prescribed antacids. She was not relieved of her symptom and met the physician two weeks later when she was asked to take anthelmintics. A month or two later another physician examined her, found ascites and a mass abdomen. Further investigations confirmed ovarian cancer.

Therefore one should have a high index of suspicion whenever elderly women present with a complaint of dyspepsia.

✤ Loss of appetite could signify cancer anywhere in the body but especially of the gastrointestinal tract.

✤ One should ask specifically about hematemesis and melena especially in those suspected to be suffering from ovarian cancer as it may be secondary to cancer in the stomach. Similarly, symptoms of carcinoma colon such as increasing constipation or alternating diarrhea and constipation, should be elicited because ovarian and colonic cancer may co-exist.

Alterations in bowel habits may also be attributed to pressure of tumours on the rectum.

✤ Urinary symptoms like increased frequency may be due to fibroids situated on the anterior wall of the uterus. A posterior cervical fibroid often gives rise to retention of urine. Hematuria is a feature of bladder cancer.

✤ Fever, especially in the evening, could be due to an encysted tuberculous peritonitis or tubo-ovarian masses of tuberculous origin. High spiking fever is associated with a tubo-ovarian abscess. Sometimes patients with embryonal tumour may present with fever.

✤ Jaundice is a manifestation of liver metastasis and may occur in case of ovarian cancer.

✤ History of infertility is more frequently associated with fibroids than with ovarian tumours.

✤ Efforts should be made to find out if the patient suffered from tuberculosis or pelvic inflammatory disease in the past. This would be particularly relevant in suspected cases of intestinal tuberculosis and tubo-ovarian masses. If there is history of surgery suggestive of myomectomy, the mass currently investigated may be a recurrent fibroid.

❖ Fibroids are sometimes seen to occur among siblings, in mother and daughter or maternal aunt and niece. There is a genetic risk for site-specific cancer like ovarian cancer. Ovarian cancer could occur more frequently among women with a family history of colonic, endometrial and breast cancer.

PHYSICAL EXAMINATION

General examination
General examination must be performed with particular attention to the following:

❖ Cachexia is present in ovarian cancer or very large benign ovarian tumours. An ill child with fever may have an embryonal tumour.

❖ Jaundice may be present in malignant ovarian tumours.

❖ While examining the breasts, one must look for changes suggestive of pregnancy or presence of a lump that could be a fibroadenoma or cancer.

❖ Enlargement of lymph nodes in the cervical region suggests tuberculosis.

❖ Palpable left supraclavicular node is indicative of cancer ovary.

Abdominal examination
Inspection
A note must be made as to whether the abdominal distension is localised or generalised. The umbilicus could be displaced upwards by a mass arising from the pelvis; it could be everted in the presence of ascites. A record should be made about the movements of the abdomen during respiration as they may be restricted by a large mass or by inflammation.

Palpation
a. **Mass in the hypogastrium**

i. The urinary bladder forms a globular swelling in the hypogastrium. If a patient has difficulty in passing urine, especially in the postpartum period or in elderly women, the bladder must be catheterised. There have been occasions when the 'ovarian cyst' has disappeared on catheterisation of the bladder.

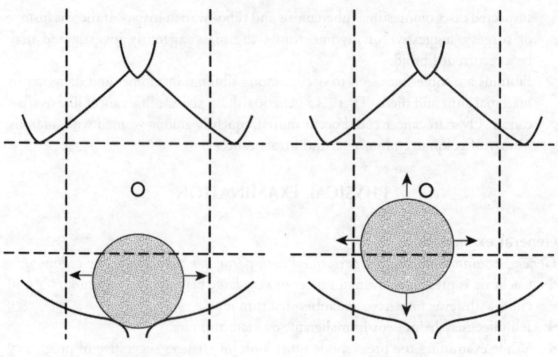

Fig. 32.1 Uterine mass   Fig. 32.2 Ovarian mass

Fig. 32.3 Mesenteric cyst

ii. Two common causes of uterine enlargement are pregnancy and fibroid uterus. In pregnancy, the uterus is uniformly enlarged and internal or external ballotment can be elicited. Uterine enlargement due to a fibroid is mostly irregular and the extent of enlargement is variable, from just above the symphysis pubis to well above umbilicus. The surface is lobulated, consistency is firm and the mass is mobile in the horizontal axis (Fig. 32.1) due its attachment to vagina. Other causes of uterine enlargement are hydatidiform mole, where the consistency is 'doughy'; uniform cystic enlargement occurs in pyometra. In case of endometrial cancer or metropathia hemorrhagica, the uterus is rarely enlarged enough to be palpable in the abdomen.

iii. Ovarian tumours—The tumours arising from the ovary are mostly cystic, have a long pedicle, are therefore mobile, and can be lifted out of the pelvis. In other words, the lower margin of the tumour is palpable. Mobility of the mass can be elicited in both the horizontal and vertical axes (Fig. 32.2). If the tumour has undergone torsion or is infected, and in cases of malignancy, mobility could be restricted.

iv. Encysted tuberculous peritonitis may be mistaken for an ovarian tumour. It is not mobile and is usually resonant on percussion due to surrounding bowel loops.

v. The mesenteric cyst is not located in the hypogastrium. However, it may have to be differentiated from a large ovarian cyst which has grown into the abdomen. The mobility of the mesenteric cyst will be at right angles to the line of attachment of the mesentery (Fig. 32.3).

vi. A hydatid cyst could present as a non-mobile mass, dull on percussion.

b. **Mass in the right iliac region**

i. An ovarian tumour is not always restricted to the side from which it arises unless there is torsion or a short pedicle. Quite often, an ovarian tumour presents as a mass in the hypogastrium.

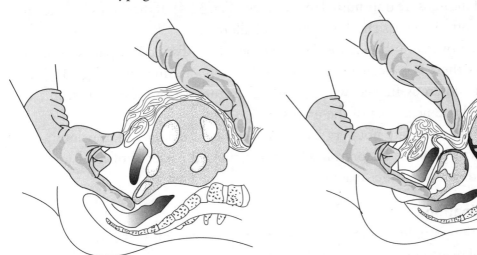

Fig. 32.4 Movements of mass transmitted to cervix (uterine mass)   **Fig. 32.5 A groove is felt between the uterus and the mass (adnexal mass)**

ii. A tubo-ovarian mass is almost always inflammatory in nature; endometriosis of the ovary can give rise to such a mass.

iii. A subserous pedunculated fibroid is mobile and firm in consistency.

iv. Carcinoma of the fallopian tube is rare and is seen in elderly women who complain of blood-stained watery discharge per vaginum.

v. Appendicular lump—This develops a few days after an attack of acute appendicitis; the location of the mass corresponds to the position of the appendix.

vi. Enlargement of iliac group of nodes—This is due to malignancies.

vii. An ileocecal mass is usually due to tuberculosis and cancer; it is fixed in the right iliac fossa.

c. **Mass in the left iliac region**

The mass could arise from the *left ovary* and/or the *fallopian tube*. Carcinoma sigmoid colon is implied in a not very large mass with restricted mobility.

Abdominal palpation must be performed to check for other masses, especially omental mass in case of ovarian cancer. Liver, spleen and kidneys should be palpated.

Percussion must be performed to ascertain the presence of ascites.

Vaginal examination

This examination is crucial in helping to differentiate a uterine mass from an adnexal mass. On bimanual examination, a uterine mass is continuous with the cervix and the movements of the mass are transmitted to the cervix (Fig. 32.4). If the uterus is uniformly enlarged and soft, one must check for internal ballotment.

In case of an ovarian tumour, the mass can be felt as distinctly separate from the uterus, unless there has been malignant infiltration or infection (Fig. 32.5). A pedunculated subserous fibroid will also be felt separate from the uterus, but the consistency is the same as that of the uterus.

Tubo-ovarian masses are not very large; they are firm, tender and are close to the uterus. However, previous history of pelvic infection and presence of fever and pain distinguishes them from other masses.

Rectal examination

This examination is useful to check if the uterus has been pushed posteriorly by a mass. In case of malignancy, there could be metastatic nodules in the pouch of Douglas.

INVESTIGATIONS

The information obtained from a good history and physical examination will help to make a diagnosis in more than 60 per cent of cases. Investigations should be selected to confirm the nature of the mass whenever necessary and to carry out a detailed study of the tumour.

Ultrasonography is indicated in the following situations:

❖ To determine the anatomical origin of the mass, where the clinical findings are ambiguous

❖ To determine presence of a fetus to confirm pregnancy

❖ Whenever myomectomy is planned, as in case of fibroid with infertility, to assess the number of fibroids and their encroachment on the endometrial cavity

❖ Hydatidiform mole shows a typical 'snow-storm' appearance

❖ In case of ovarian tumours, the malignant nature can be determined by the presence of thick septae, papillary excrescences and variegated appearance.

❖ It is essential to study the liver, spleen and kidneys. For example, the kidney may be hydronephrotic in case of very large fibroids or ovarian tumours.

TREATMENT

 What interventional strategies should one adopt?

In most cases of mass lower abdomen, the intervention is essentially surgical. Fibroids are treated by myomectomy in younger women and in older women by hysterectomy (see Chapter 29). Asymptomatic fibroids in perimenopausal women, need to be operated if the uterine enlargement is more than 14 weeks pregnant uterus' size.

Surgery for ovarian tumours in younger women consists of ovariectomy/ovariotomy; ideally a frozen section report should be obtained to rule out malignancy. In women, especially those above 40 years of age, a thorough exploration of the abdomen and pelvis, and peritoneal cytology should be followed by ipsilateral ovariectomy, contralateral oophorectomy, hysterectomy and omentectomy where indicated.

Key points

1. A distended bladder should be excluded by catheterisation, if necessary.
2. Pregnancy should always be excluded in a woman of reproductive age group presenting with mass abdomen.
3. Menorrhagia and dysmenorrhea are characteristic of fibroid uterus.
4. Presence of fever is indicative of masses of infective origin, especially tuberculosis.
5. A high index of suspicion for ovarian cancer is warranted if an elderly woman complains of dyspepsia.

CHAPTER 33

Acute pain lower abdomen

ASHA OUMACHIGUI

Acute pain lower abdomen may be defined as a condition where a patient presents with severe abdominal pain and other symptoms that suggest a disease which could be life-threatening, but that do not necessarily warrant immediate surgical intervention. The underlying pathology could be in the gastrointestinal, urinary or genital system. A diagnosis should be made at the earliest, and immediate therapeutic intervention should be instituted in order to avoid a fatal outcome. This is particularly true of ruptured ectopic pregnancy which accounts for a significant number of maternal deaths.

Objectives

At the end of this chapter, the reader should be able to

- ❑ Define acute pain lower abdomen.
- ❑ Enumerate diseases responsible for the condition.
- ❑ List the clinical features of common causes of acute pain lower abdomen.
- ❑ List relevant laboratory investigations to confirm the diagnosis.
- ❑ Refer the patient appropriately, without delay, after instituting immediate therapy.
- ❑ Outline a plan of management for the common conditions.

CLINICAL SCENARIO

A 28-year-old woman presents with severe lower abdominal pain of four hours duration.

HISTORY

The history should be elicited particularly with two points in mind:

i.   A 'high index' of suspicion of ectopic pregnancy in a woman in the reproductive age group.

ii. A young woman can suffer from an acute pain lower abdomen due to diseases that affect systems other than the reproductive system. Diagnosis is challenging if she is pregnant.

 What questions should be asked to gain a better understanding of the case?

All details related to pain should be elicited.

❖ Mode of onset – The pain starts suddenly in ectopic pregnancy with tubal perforation, hollow viscus perforation, colic, torsion and volvulus. In acute appendicitis, the pain is not acute at onset unless there is obstruction of the appendiceal lumen.

❖ Time of onset – Pain, abdominal or pelvic is the most constant feature of ectopic pregnancy (95 per cent). The onset is not related to any particular time of the day

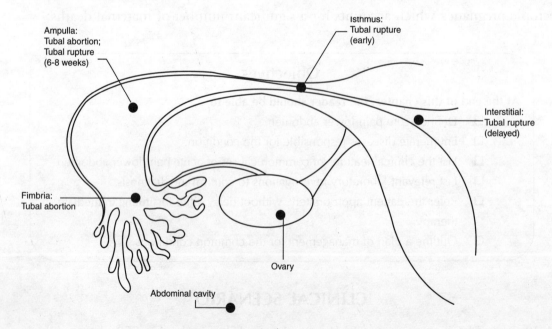

Fig. 33.1 Sites and outcome of ectopic pregnancy

or night. The clinical presentation depends on the mode of termination of the ectopic pregnancy which is closely related to the site of implantation in the fallopian tube (Fig. 33.1).

If there is rupture of tubal pregnancy, the patient is struck down by an attack of pain. This is caused by damage to the tubal wall by the eroding trophoblast, just as it occurs in the uterus in the formation of the intervillous space. The uterus has a thick muscle wall and well-formed decidua, but in the tube, the thin sheets of circular and longitudinal muscle fibres are soon destroyed.

This type of 'fulminant' tubal rupture is uncommon. In most cases, premonitory symptoms are likely to have been present for hours or even days before the woman has sudden massive hemorrhage.

The more common presentation is one where the woman has abdominal uneasiness or chronic pain for a few days, followed by an acute attack.

❖ The duration of pain is variable in ectopic pregnancy, twisted ovarian cyst, acute salpingitis or appendicitis.

❖ The pain may be anywhere in the abdomen if there is hemoperitoneum. In case of a pelvic hematocele, the pain may be localised to the pelvis or it may be in one of the iliac fossae if there is a tubal mole.

❖ Shifting pain is characteristic of appendicitis; the pain is initially around the umbilicus and later shifts to the right iliac fossa.

❖ Radiation of pain—Initially the pain is localised to the region of the affected organ, but later, with spreading peritonitis, the patient complains of pain all over the abdomen.

❖ Referred pain—The pain is said to be 'referred' when it is felt at some other region having the same segmental innervation as the site of the lesion. The diaphragm is supplied by the phrenic nerves C3, C4 and C5. The cutaneous nerves from the same segments supply the skin over the shoulder; blood, pus, bile or gas in the peritoneal cavity can irritate the undersurface of the diaphragm giving rise to pain in the shoulder. This symptom is characteristic of disturbed ectopic pregnancy which is associated with hemoperitoneum.

❖ Character of the pain—The pain is excruciating in ectopic pregnancy, twisted ovarian cyst and acute salpingitis. Colicky pain points to spasm or obstruction of a hollow organ.

In some cases of ectopic pregnancy, the pain may be very acute in the initial phases, settling down to abdominal uneasiness to become acute whenever there is hemorrhage.

1. Factors relieving or aggravating pain—Colicky pain is relieved by pressure to some extent. In conditions like pelvic abscess, hematocele and ureteric colic, pain is aggravated by micturition or coughing. Once generalised peritonitis sets in, any movement makes the pain more severe.

2. Fever—A rise in temperature is recorded in cases of urinary tract infection (UTI), acute salpingitis, acute appendicitis, pelvic abscess and red degeneration of fibroid. It is conspicuously absent in cases of disturbed ectopic pregnancy.

3. Vomiting is a constant symptom of gastrointestinal disorders. A number of patients suffering from acute appendicitis may complain of nausea and vomiting. In acute salpingitis and ectopic pregnancy, vomiting is secondary to generalised peritonitis. Vomiting may also accompany severe pain.

4. Bowel symptoms—In pelvic abscess, hematocele and pelvic appendicitis, irritation of the rectum leads to ineffectual straining at stools, tenesmus and mucus diarrhea.

5. Painful, frequent attempts at micturition indicate UTI or a stone in the bladder or the lower end of ureter. Pelvic peritonitis due to ectopic pregnancy or pelvic abscess can give rise to similar symptoms.

6. Menstrual symptoms
   ❖ Amenorrhea—A short period of amenorrhea (6–8 weeks) could be due to an ectopic pregnancy. However, in about 25 per cent of cases there may be no history of missed period. It is important to elicit at this stage, the character of the last menstrual period, for example scanty bleeding. Severe abdominal pain, cyclical to begin with, and primary amenorrhea point to hematometra (cryptomenorrhea).
   ❖ History of pain associated with menstruation suggests dysmenorrhea.

7. Vaginal bleeding—In ectopic pregnancy, the vaginal bleeds are small, unlike in disturbed intrauterine pregnancy, where bleeding is profuse. In ectopic pregnancy, the degree of pallor noted on general examination is out of proportion to the amount of bleeding. Blood-stained discharge may be noted in cases of twisted ovarian cyst.

8. A history suggestive of pelvic inflammatory disease, infertility and any operation on the fallopian tube, especially recanalisation, is very relevant when ectopic pregnancy is suspected.

Independent factors consistently shown to increase the risk of tubal pregnancy are:
* Previous proved pelvic inflammatory disease
* Previous tubal pregnancy
* Current IUCD use
* Previous tubal surgery, especially recanalisation

EXAMINATION

General physical examination

A patient suffering from acute pain lower abdomen will appear ill. Presence of moderate to severe pallor points to internal hemorrhage, most often due to a disturbed ectopic pregnancy. However, it is prudent to remember that in India and other developing countries, moderate to severe anemia is fairly common in women of reproductive age.

There is fever and tachycardia in acute appendicitis and acute salpingitis and also in other conditions, when peritonitis sets in.

In ectopic pregnancy, response to moderate hemorrhage may range from no change in pulse and blood pressure, to a mild tachycardia or a vasovagal response with bradycardia and hypotension. Since most women suffering from ectopic pregnancy are young, a rise in pulse rate and fall in blood pressure will occur only if hypovolemia becomes significant.

Abdominal examination

An *inspection* of the abdomen may reveal varying degrees of distension depending on the extent of peritonitis. A localised distension may be visible in the lower abdomen in case of a twisted ovarian cyst.

The patient's confidence should be gained before beginning *palpation*. The examination should be performed gently. The whole abdomen must be palpated to appreciate muscle guarding (involuntary muscular rigidity). The presence of this feature is indicative of underlying peritonitis. The rigidity may be localised in early stages of twisted ovarian cyst, ectopic pregnancy or appendicitis.

A lump in one of the iliac fossae is suggestive of twisted ovarian cyst; an appendicular lump will be felt in the right iliac fossa. A fibroid with red degeneration presents as a mass in the hypogastrium.

Percussion helps to elicit shifting dullness, which indicates the presence of free fluid

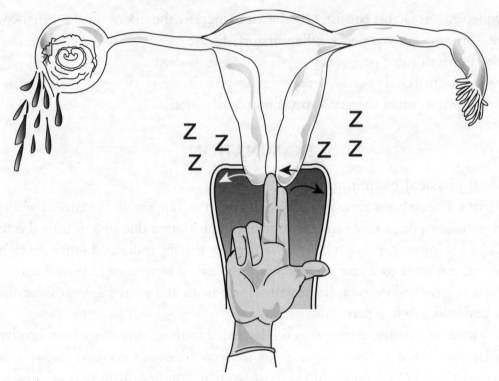

Fig. 33.2 Tenderness on movement of cervix

in the peritoneal cavity. There are a number of conditions such as ruptured ectopic pregnancy and perforation of peptic ulcer where free fluid accumulates in the peritoneal cavity.

Obliteration of liver dullness indicates free gas under the diaphragm and occurs in perforation of the gastrointestinal tract.

Auscultation will reveal absence of bowel sounds whenever there is paralytic ileus secondary to peritonitis.

Pelvic examination

A vaginal speculum examination gives an idea about the nature of bleeding or discharge through the cervical os. A small quantity of bleeding suggests extrauterine pregnancy, while purulent discharge is suggestive of pelvic infection or septic abortion.

Complications of abortions due to unskilled interference are still common in developing countries. Therefore, the vagina and the cervix should be inspected for the presence of injuries.

Bimanual vaginal examination—The outstanding feature of an ectopic pregnancy with recently effused blood is: marked tenderness on palpation of the vaginal vault or on gently moving the cervix, a tenderness which often prevents adequate palpation of the adnexae. The tenderness has been described as 'yelling tenderness' characteristic of acute salpingitis, more applicable to a recently disturbed ectopic gestation (Fig. 33.2).

This finding in conjunction with pallor and features of hypovolemia, calls for immediate laparotomy. If facilities for laparotomy are not available, the patient must be referred to the nearest hospital after instituting resuscitative measures.

A pelvic mass measuring 5–15 cm may be palpable in 20–50 per cent of patients. The mass is usually a peritubal hematocele and is soft in consistency and 'elastic'. However, with accumulation of blood in the tubal lumen, the mass may feel firm.

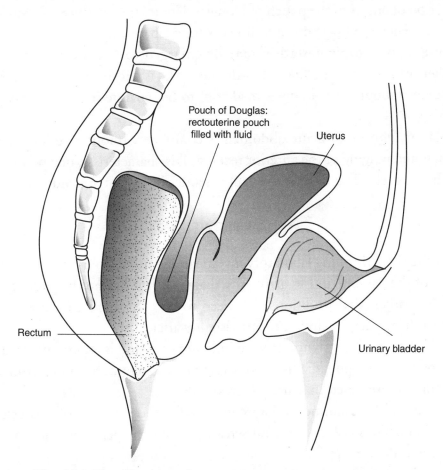

Fig. 33.3 Blood/pus in pelvic cavity: sagittal section of pelvis

Sometimes, there may be a diffuse swelling/fullness in the pouch of Douglas. If not treated at this stage, there is an increasing accumulation of blood leading to the formation of a pelvic hematocele large enough to be palpable per abdomen.

At this stage, culdocentesis may be performed in order to detect a hemoperitoneum or a pelvic abscess (Fig. 33.3). Culdocentesis is a simple technique—the cervix is pulled towards the symphysis pubis with a tenaculum and a long 16–18 gauge needle is inserted through the posterior fornix into the pouch of Douglas. Failure of aspirated blood to clot is compatible with the diagnosis of disturbed ectopic gestation. However, failure to obtain blood from the pouch of Douglas does not always rule out the diagnosis of hemoperitoneum because adhesions in the pelvis may prevent the blood from reaching the pouch of Douglas.

Aspiration of pus from the pouch of Douglas denotes the presence of a pelvic abscess. Presence of generalised peritonitis will necessitate laparotomy.

The uterus in ectopic gestation may be enlarged to 6–8 weeks' size.

Another situation where a fairly well-defined mass is felt through one of the fornices is an ovarian tumour. The uterus is made out to be separate from the mass, and is of normal size.

No examination of an acute abdomen is complete without a *rectal examination*. Tenderness and bulging of the anterior rectal wall is characteristic of a pelvic abscess or a pelvic hematocele. The right rectal wall is tender in case of appendicitis.

INVESTIGATIONS

The objectives of performing laboratory investigations are twofold—to assess the general condition of the patient, and to arrive at a diagnosis if it has not been done so far.

As stated earlier, the conditions that need to be confirmed are ectopic gestation, acute appendicitis, acute salpingitis or twisted ovarian cyst.

1. Blood—Leukocytosis is indicative of inflammation and is an important clue in the diagnosis of acute appendicitis, acute salpingitis and septic abortion. Serum bilirubin and amylase are raised in acute pancreatitis.
2. Urine should be examined microscopically for the presence of pus cells besides sugar and albumin. A culture and sensitivity must be performed if more than 10 pus cells/HPF are seen.
3. Vaginal or cervical swab, and pus obtained on culdocentesis must be subjected to

Gram stain and culture and sensitivity.

4. An empty uterine cavity on *transvaginal sonography,* and serum β hCG levels of 1000–2000 mIU/ml are said to confirm an ectopic gestation. Ultrasonography is also useful in the detection of ovarian cyst, disturbed intrauterine pregnancy and collection of fluid in the pelvis.

TREATMENT

 What are the principles of treatment?

If the general condition of the patient so warrants, immediate resuscitative measures must be instituted even before a diagnosis is made. Conditions like disturbed ectopic pregnancy, twisted ovarian tumour and acute appendicitis require surgical intervention. Medical management is resorted to in case of acute PID unless complicated by peritonitis or a pelvic abscess. Acute urinary infections are treated with appropriate antibiotics.

Key points

1. In a patient suffering from acute pain lower abdomen, a meticulous history is mandatory.
2. Careful general physical, abdominal and bimanual examinations are invaluable.
3. In women of reproductive age group with acute lower abdominal pain, one must have a high index of suspicion for ectopic pregnancy.
4. Acute lower abdominal pain associated with fever is most likely due to UTI, pelvic infection or acute appendicitis.
5. A woman could be pregnant and suffer from nongynecological causes of acute abdominal pain.

CHAPTER 34

Chronic problems of the breast

N. ANANTHAKRISHNAN

Women may present with one or more of the problems in relation to the breast such as a) lump in the breast, b) pain in the breast, c) discharge from the nipple or d) a fear of breast cancer (cancerphobia). These presenting symptoms may occur separately or in combination. Together they account for more than 90 per cent of chronic breast problems in women. A careful history and a meticulous physical examination is important in making a tentative diagnosis so that management can be appropriately planned.

Objectives

At the end of this chapter, the reader should be able to
- ❏ Obtain appropriate history from patient with a chronic breast problem.
- ❏ Carry out physical examination understanding the relevance of various findings.
- ❏ Order appropriate investigations to arrive at a diagnosis so that further management can be planned.

HISTORY

 What are the points to be considered in the history?

1. There may be a history of early menarche, a long delay before the first child, nulliparity or a delayed menopause in patients with breast cancer. There is no definite proof that lactation protects from breast cancer.

2. ***Age*** is an important factor. Fibroadenomas of the breast occur usually between the age of 12 and 35 years. It is unusual for fibroadenomas to occur for the first time in premenopausal or perimenopausal women. A carcinoma may occur at any age. The usual age of occurrence is after 35 years. However, in women with a strong family history of breast cancer, the onset may be much earlier, even in the twenties. Mammary dysplasia (fibroadenosis) occurs in women in the reproductive age group. A discharge from the nipple starting after menopause is an ominous symptom which may point to cancer.

3. ***Pain***—Malignancy and fibroadenomas of the breast are usually painless. If *pain* is present, one should enquire whether it is cyclical or noncyclical. Cyclical pain is maximal in the premenstrual phase and is probably related to progestrone excess. Cyclical pain is almost always due to benign causes such as mammary dysplasia. Noncyclical pain may be due to inflammatory lesions, traumatic fat necrosis or occasionally due to causes in the underlying chest wall, such as costochondritis. Pain due to costochondritis is well localised to the affected costo-chondral junction.

4. ***Discharge from the nipple***—Milky discharge is found in galactoceles or galactorrhea due to hormonal imbalance in nonlactating women. A serous or greenish discharge may be seen in mammary dysplasia. It is usually bilateral and is associated with cyclical pain. Blood-stained discharge is more serious and may indicate a ductal papilloma or a ductal carcinoma.

5. ***A lump*** in the breast is by far the most common presentation. Most lumps are noticed casually while having a bath or because of associated pain. A history of blunt injury may be present in traumatic fat necrosis. The rate of growth may be gradual in benign and slow growing malignancies, whereas it is rapid in inflammatory carcinomas. Bilateral or multiple lumps are more common in fibroadenomas or mammary dysplasia. Occasionally invasive lobular carcinoma may present with bilateral lump.

6. ***Eczematous changes*** in the nipple, particularly in the absence of itching and especially if unilateral may indicate Paget's disease of the breast. *If retraction* of the nipple is present, one should enquire whether it is of recent or remote onset. Remote retraction of nipple present from adolescence is usually developmental and a history of lactational problems in the past may be obtained. Recent retraction is most commonly due to a carcinoma. Occasionally retraction may be seen in tuberculous mastitis, subareolar mastitis or traumatic fat necrosis.

7. Presentation of breast cancer with symptoms of metastatic disease such as hemoptysis or dyspnea due to pulmonary secondaries, hepatomegaly or bone pain are rare.

   A family history of breast cancer in the mother, maternal aunt, maternal grandmother or sisters should be taken. Patients with a strong family history usually have an earlier age of onset of malignancy.

PHYSICAL EXAMINATION

It is necessary to examine the patient from the top of the neck to the waist, and examine both breasts. Inspection of the breast must be carried out with the patient in the following positions:

❖ Sitting with the arms by the side
❖ Leaning forward at 45°
❖ Hyperabducting the arms so that they touch the ears
❖ Supine with a soft thin pillow under the ipsilateral chest.

Leaning forwards demonstrates tethering to the underlying muscles or chest wall. Hyperabduction often demonstrates tethering of skin or *peau d'orange* which is not obvious with the arms by the side. The best position for palpation is the last one, in which the breast tissue is spread out thinly over the chest wall and palpation of small lumps is easier particularly in a large breast.

Inspection

The points to be noted on inspection are:

❖ Size and symmetry of the breasts is often lost in a large benign or malignant tumour.
❖ Position of the nipple: infiltration of the lactiferous ducts by a malignant tumour may cause retraction and a shift of the nipple towards the tumour.
❖ Appearance and size of the areola should be noted. The areola may be expanded in patients with a large central tumour.
❖ Prominent cutaneous vessels indicate a vascular neoplasm. Prominence of veins in the parasternal area with a flow away from the midline may indicate blockage of the internal mammary veins due to enlarged internal mammary nodes.
❖ Retraction of the skin is due to shortening of the ligaments of Cooper either by an inflammatory process or more commonly, a malignant tumour. *Peau d'orange* is due to blockage of the subcuticular lymphatics by tumour deposit leading to edema

of the skin. However, the mouths of the skin appendages such as the hair follicles or the apocrine glands remain tethered to the dermis giving an 'orange peel' appearance to the skin.

♣ Cutaneous nodules separated from the primary lump are indications of locally advanced breast cancer.

♣ One should look carefully for localised lumps. Unless large, these may be missed on inspection. If overlying ulceration is present, it may be due to infiltration of the skin due to carcinoma or stretch necrosis as in cystosarcoma phylloides. A stretch necrotic ulcer usually has undermined edges. The tumour which forms the floor may protrude above the surrounding skin. In case of infiltration due to a carcinoma the margins of the ulcer would be rolled out.

♣ The axillae, supraclavicular fossae and the opposite breast should be inspected for visible swellings.

Palpation

Start with palpating the uninvolved breast, first with the palmar surface of the fingers for detecting lumpiness or lumps and then with the pulp of the thumb and fingers for detailed assessment. The central segment and all four quadrants including the axillary tail should be systematically palpated. One should proceed from the periphery to the centre to note whether any nipple discharge is produced. Important facts to be noted on palpation are:

1. Tenderness and temperature: These are more common with inflammatory swellings.
2. Whether the whole breast is involved or only one or two segments by a palpable abnormality.
3. Diffuse nodularity is better felt with the pulp rather than the flat of the fingers. This finding is characteristically seen in fibroadenosis.
4. If a definite lump is palpable then the following should be noted:
   a. Site
   b. Shape
   c. Margins—The margins of an inflammatory mass are usually diffuse while they are well defined in a neoplasm. The margin is regular or smooth in benign swellings and irregular in malignancy.
   d. Surface—The surface may be smooth in a breast cyst or a fibroadenoma. It is usually uneven in malignancy.

e. Consistency—Most carcinomas are hard, with the exception of an inflammatory carcinoma or a medullary carcinoma which may be soft to firm; fibroadenomas are usually firm.

f. Intramammary mobility—A fibroadenoma, and occasionally a cyst in the breast, may be displaced from one segment to another without dragging the surrounding breast tissue along with it. Fibroadenoma with such mobility is referred to as a 'breast mouse'. Significant intramammary mobility is not present in malignancy.

g. Transillumination and fluctuation have no role in conventional clinical examination of the breast.

h. Tethering or fixation to skin with inability to pinch or move the skin on the underlying mass is a feature of malignancy.

i. Fixity to underlying structures: Three muscles underlie the breast: the pectoralis major related to the central and upper quadrants, the serratus anterior to the lower lateral quadrant and the rectus abdominis and external oblique related to the lower inner quadrant. The mobility of the lump on these muscles should be tested with the muscles relaxed holding the base of the lump between the pulp of the fingers, and again with the muscles contracted. Reduction or loss of mobility in the direction of the muscle fibres is important and indicates fixation. A lump which is fixed to the chest wall would have no movement even with the underlying muscles relaxed. Assessment of fixation to fascia is by a process of elimination. A breast lump which does not fall forwards on leaning but is not demonstrably fixed to underlying muscle on examination is fixed to the pectoral fascia. Fixation to fascia or underlying pectoral muscle does not affect staging. Fixation to the serratus anterior is considered fixation to chest wall and the lesion is described as T_4.

Palpation of lymph nodes—The lymph nodes draining the breast are the pectoral or anterior axillary, the central axillary, the subscapular or posterior axillary, the apical, the internal mammary and supraclavicular nodes.

Internal mammary nodes are best detected on CT scan. When large, there may be parasternal dullness in the upper 2–3 intercostal spaces.

Anterior axillary nodes are best felt with the ipsilateral forearm resting on the examinee's forearm. The lymph nodes are felt with the fingers behind the pectoral muscles and the thumb in front. Central axillary nodes are felt by inserting the hand as high as possible in the axilla and moving the palmar surface of the fingers downward, along the chest wall.

Posterior axillary nodes are felt from behind the patient with the fingers in front of the posterior axillary fold and the thumb behind it. Apical axillary nodes are difficult to feel. The hand is introduced deep into the axilla and counterpressure is applied with the other hand in the supraclavicular fossa. The supraclavicular nodes are felt from behind the patient by inserting the fingers behind the clavicle and rolling the tissues over the first rib.

A note should be made of the number, size, consistency of lymph nodes and presence or absence of matting.

SYSTEMIC EXAMINATION

Examination of the breast is incomplete without systemic examination. One should check for rib and spinal tenderness, evidence of pleural effusion, mediastinal widening, hepatomegaly, upper paraaortic lymph nodes, ascites and ovarian enlargement due to malignant deposits.

INVESTIGATIONS

The principal aims of investigations in a patient with a chronic breast problem are:
* Confirm the diagnosis
* If malignant, assess extent of spread
* Assess fitness for treatment

Investigations for confirming diagnosis are:
1. Fine needle aspiration cytology (FNAC) is by far the best method of confirming the diagnosis. It is accurate and sensitive. A false positive and false negative diagnosis of malignancy is rare. Occasionally, an indeterminate FNAC may require a core needle biopsy for confirming diagnosis. Sometimes, in suspicious cases where FNAC and core needle biopsy are inconclusive, an excision biopsy for paraffin section can be done. Currently, frozen sections are rarely used to diagnose breast lesions. Cytological evaluation of the discharge from the nipple may yield diagnostic material.
2. A chest x-ray is mandatory to look for pleural effusion, pulmonary secondaries or

mediastinal widening. A more penetrated view is required to look for deposits in the ribs.

3. Ultrasonography of the abdomen is indicated to detect liver secondaries, ascites and ovarian metastasis. Upper paraaortic nodes are better seen with a CT scan.

4. A skeletal survey is not indicated routinely. In case of bone pain or bony tenderness, a skiagram of the affected part is taken. Bone scan is indicated in advanced breast carcinoma and in patients with x-ray negative bone pain. Secondary deposits appear as hot spots on the bone scan.

5. *Mammography* is generally to be used only for screening purposes and not in the work up of a patient with a breast lump. Its use as a diagnostic investigation is limited to the following situations:
   ❖ An indistinct mass in a large breast
   ❖ Vague masses after previous surgery
   ❖ Evaluation of the opposite breast particularly in invasive lobular carcinoma
   ❖ For tumour localisation for stereotaxic biopsy
   ❖ In patients with cancerphobia and a strong family history of breast cancer
   A malignant mass has indistinct crenated margins, may show edema of the overlying skin, distortion of the normal ductal architecture or clustered microcalcification. A benign mass will be well defined with regular smooth margins.

6. Occasionally contrast is injected into the mamillary ducts (mamillography) for evaluating patients with discharge from the nipple. Intraductal filling defects may indicate an intraductal tumour.

7. Sentinel node biopsy. Recently attempts have been made using either dyes or radio-isotopes to locate the first lymphatic filter of the breast. After localisation, these nodes are excised for histological examination.

8. Examination of the excised lump in malignancy, for estrogen and progesterone receptors is important for prognosis and for choice of therapy.

Principles of treatment

1. Cyclical mastalgia often associated with dysmenorrhea may respond to hormoral therapy. Noncyclical mastalgia requires reassurance, breast support and occasionally use of analgesics.

2. Patients with nipple discharge and a palpable lump should have therapy based on the nature of the lump. Other patients with discharge localised to one duct orifice,

can undergo excision of the particular ductal segment (microdochectomy) and further treatment after histological examination of the specimen.

3. Patients with diffuse nodularity and benign on FNAC findings only require reassurance, baseline mammography and periodic re-examination.
4. Single fibroadenomas can be excised. Multiple fibroadenomas, in young women can be treated expectantly. Occasionally some lesions may undergo regression.
5. Patients with breast cancer require appropriate therapy depending on the stage of the disease.

Key points

1. Lump in the breast, pain or nipple discharge account for a vast majority of presenting symptoms in the breast.
2. A good history goes a long way in narrowing down the possibilities.
3. Loss of intramammary mobility, irregular margin, tethering of skin, fixity to deeper structures, hardness and palpable regional nodes point towards malignancy.
4. FNAC remains the most useful initial investigation. Core needle biopsy is indicated in those instances where FNAC is inconclusive.
5. Mammography has its best application as a screening investigation and for evaluating indistinct masses in a bulky breast. It is also useful for follow up of the opposite breast after ipsilateral mastectomy.

CHAPTER 35

Inability to conceive

GITA RAJAGOPALAN

To procreate is one of the inherent needs of human beings. It is often considered an important goal of marriage. Inability to conceive may have several social and psychological consequences. Often, the woman is held responsible for this. Therefore, she is brought to the gynecologist for treatment. It is necessary to remember that either partner may contribute to this problem. Inability to conceive is called infertility. If the failure to conceive is absolute, it is called sterility.

Objectives

At the end of this chapter, the reader should be able to

❑ Decide when a couple who fails to achieve pregnancy needs to be investigated.

❑ Understand the aims of investigation of an infertile couple.

❑ Appreciate the need to see the couple rather than the female partner alone.

❑ Elicit relevant history from both the partners.

❑ Perform a clinical examination of the woman and the man.

❑ Select relevant investigations and interpret the results.

❑ Outline the plan of treatment.

❑ Counsel the couple about the prognosis.

CLINICAL SCENARIO

A 20-year-old woman who has been married for one year consults a gynecologist because she has not conceived.

About 85–90 per cent of women conceive within the first year of marriage if they have been having intercourse without protection. Inability of a couple to achieve pregnancy after one year of regular and unprotected coitus is called infertility. Some experts believe it is better to wait for two years before diagnosing it as 'infertility'. If the girl is in her teens, it is prudent to wait till she is at least 20 years old. However, if the woman is 30 years old or more, it may be worthwhile to investigate even after six months of regular unprotected intercourse since the fertility of women declines, starting from the thirties.

In every case, the woman may be examined before explaining the appropriate time for the investigation for infertility. The two important aims of infertility work up are to find out the cause of infertility and to explain the prognosis after investigations, to the couple.

HISTORY

 What questions should be asked to gain a better understanding of the case?

The questions asked are very personal and at times the couple may not be forthcoming in answering them. It may be worthwhile to meet them frequently, establish a good rapport and obtain the information gradually.

In the female partner, one should enquire about age of menarche, duration and regularity of menstrual cycles, amount of menstrual flow and presence of dysmenorrhea. Regular menstrual cycles with dysmenorrhea indicate regular ovulation.

Any past history of pregnancy, its outcome, and occurrence of abnormal pregnancies should be noted. If a pregnancy has occurred earlier and the couple is currently unable to achieve pregnancy, this is **secondary infertility**.

Past medical history should include history of tuberculosis and mumps. History of any abdominal surgery like appendicectomy or pelvic surgery like D and C, induced abortion should be asked for. One must ask for sexually transmitted diseases particularly gonococcal infections and other reproductive tract infections. Intolerance to cold, constipation and lethargy indicate hypothyroidism. Headaches, diplopia or vomiting may point to a pituitary cause. Abnormal hair growth can occur in PCOS and adrenal disorders. Family history of infertility or amenorrhea is also relevant.

In the male partner, the age, occupation, particularly the working environment, and whether the job involves frequent travelling should be ascertained.

History of mumps, tuberculosis or filarial infections should be enquired into. Diabetes may cause autonomic disorders resulting in impotence. Past history of surgery for hernia, hydrocele or varicocele may affect fertility. One should elicit history of trauma to the testes. Personal habits like smoking, alcohol or drug use should also be enquired into. All these have a deleterious effect on fertility. History of premarital or extramarital contacts, and sexually transmitted diseases, particularly gonococcal infections should be obtained.

In both partners, confirm that the couple is living together. Coital history has to be tactfully obtained, if necessary by interviewing the partners repeatedly, and at times, separately. Frequency of coitus, timing in relation to fertile period, history of impotence, premature ejaculation, sexual dissatisfaction, dyspareunia or retrograde ejaculation are to be elicited.

PHYSICAL EXAMINATION

A physical examination of the woman is performed initially. In general examination, pallor, lymphadenopathy, height, weight, development of breasts, presence of galactorrhea, enlargement of thyroid gland, development of axillary and pubic hair, pattern of hair distribution and presence of abnormal hair growth should be looked for.

Hepatomegaly, splenomegaly, masses or ascites should be excluded by abdominal examination.

One should thoroughly inspect the external genitalia and note its development. There may be thick, rigid or annular hymen. The vagina may be narrow, or may go into spasm during the examination. These findings confirm coital difficulties. A speculum examination is useful in detecting discharge suggestive of trichomonal vaginitis, candidiasis or gonococcal infection.

A bimanual examination will help to confirm the normal development of the uterus and also exclude conditions like fibroid uterus, ovarian cysts or pelvic inflammatory disease. Tenderness on deep palpation or a retroverted, fixed and tender uterus may suggest the presence of endometriosis or PID.

INVESTIGATIONS

It is prudent to get a semen analysis done initially. Often the male partner may not be available or willing for any investigation. One must ensure that the male partner is normal because the investigations of the female partner are invasive and expensive. If semen analysis is found to be abnormal, it may be repeated once or twice. In case of an abnormal seminogram, the male partner should be examined.

Normal seminogram

Volume	:	2–6 ml
Count	:	20 million/ml, or 40 million/ejaculate
Motility	:	At least 50 per cent actively motile
Morphology	:	At least 30 per cent normal forms
Vitality	:	At least 75 per cent live
Pus cells	:	< 1 million/ml

Development of secondary sexual characteristics, evidence of endocrine disorders, and sexually transmitted diseases should be recorded. Examination of genitalia for phimosis, hypospadias, chordee, varicocele or undescended testes is important. The vas deferens and epididymis should be palpated for thickening, nodularity or tenderness. The testes should be palpated for their size, presence of testicular sensation or tenderness. Hydrocele and inguinal hernias should be excluded.

Depending on the clinical situation, further investigations of the male partner may be requested.

Investigation of the female partner

Investigations to assess the general condition, like hemoglobin and urinalysis are performed. Serological test for syphilis may be done. An erythrocyte sedimentation rate (ESR) and x-ray chest are useful to rule out tuberculosis. Diabetes should be excluded by testing blood glucose levels.

Specific investigations are directed towards establishing ovulation and tubal patency. Ovulation can be confirmed by a premenstrual endometrial biopsy or follicular monitoring by ultrasound. A serum progesterone level of >3 ng/ml on day 22 will also confirm ovulation. Most tests for ovulation are indirect.

Tubal patency may be established by a hysterosalpingogram. This has the additional advantage of revealing any abnormality of uterine cavity. It may also help to identify the level of tubal block.

Laparoscopy is often performed to assess tubal patency, by injecting methylene blue through the cervix and the fimbrial ends are visualised for spillage of the dye. Laparoscopy has an advantage over the hysterosalpingogram in that the tubes and ovaries can be studied. The peritoneal cavity can be inspected for presence of conditions like adhesions, endometriosis or tuberculosis. Hysteroscopy can be combined with laparoscopy.

Postcoital test and sperm penetration tests help in identifying cervical and immunological factors.

Endocrine evaluation of the woman, and occasionally her partner, may include thyroid function tests, FSH, LH, prolactin or androgen estimations.

TREATMENT

 What are the options?

In the male, if there is oligospermia, clomiphene citrate 25 mg daily, 25 days a month for 3 months may improve the semen parameters. Correction of varicocele or vasal obstruction requires surgery. Infection should be treated by a course of doxycycline 100 mg twice a day for at least 2–4 weeks.

In the woman, anovulation is treated with ovulation inducing drugs. Clomiphene citrate in doses of 50–150 mg daily may be given from day 2 to day 6 of the menstrual cycle. Dexamethasone may be useful in hyperandrogenism and bromocriptine in hyperprolactinemia, in combination with clomiphene citrate.

If treatment with clomiphene citrate is unsuccessful, gonadotrophin therapy may be considered. GnRH may help in hypothalamic failure. **All the above treatment regimens could result in ovarian hyperstimulation syndrome or multiple ovulations and there is need for careful monitoring.**

Surgical treatment is needed for peritubal adhesions, tubal block or fibroids. The prognosis depends on the cause and the extent of disease. Surgery should be performed by laparoscopy wherever possible. Polycystic ovaries may be treated with ovarian drilling or wedge resection if there is no response to medical therapy. Endometriosis may be ablated by laparoscopic electrocautery or laser vaporisation. Medical treatment of endometriosis with progestogens, danazol or GnRH agonists relieve symptoms but may not improve fertility. Genital tuberculosis should be treated with anti-tubercular drugs, but the couple must be warned about the poor prognosis.

Sperm improvement techniques like split fraction ejaculate, centrifugation, migration procedures like swim up technique or aspiration of sperm from epididymis may be combined with intrauterine insemination. This procedure may also be useful in some coital disorders.

Role of assisted reproduction techniques (ART)

In these procedures the gametes are manipulated. They involve prolonged, expensive and invasive investigations. They are useful in unexplained infertility, tubal disease and some cases of immunological infertility. The option of ART should be explained to the couple. Factors like time, expense and success rates should be made clear and the choice of ART should rest with the couple. The gynecologist should only help them to make a decision.

Role of counselling

First of all, explain to the couple the prognosis after the investigations. Often, they have difficulty in coming to terms with reality. Gentle and repeated reassurance will help. There is significant psychological stress associated with infertility and the couple should be given help to cope with it.

When a couple chooses to undergo ART, the financial implications, the success rate, and the need for prolonged, invasive monitoring should be explained so that they can be understood and accepted.

Sometimes the attending physician has to play the role of a counsellor as marital disharmony or an incongenial domestic atmosphere may be the basic cause of the problem.

For couples who have an untreatable factor or for whom repeated therapeutic interventions have been unsuccessful, adoption may be suggested. Adoption is perhaps neither commonly advised nor accepted. However, a good gynecologist can help the couple to decide on this viable option. Most couples are very reluctant initially, but repeated sessions of counselling may help them to accept adoption, which may enable them to lead a happier life. Since many couples may be unable to afford the investigations and treatment procedures, adoption is certainly a good alternative.

Key points

1.　Infertility is a problem of the couple, not of the female partner alone.
2.　The male partner may contribute directly in a third cases and indirectly in another third.
3.　Semen analysis should be done before the female partner is investigated.
4.　Premenstrual endometrial biopsy is useful for detection of ovulation and to rule out genital tuberculosis.
5.　Laparoscopy will help to evaluate tubal and peritoneal factors.
6.　Appropriate treatment including ART should be instituted.
7.　Adoption should be offered as an option when the couple fails to conceive after treatment.

CHAPTER 36

Helping clients choose contraception

A. BUPATHY

Whatever your cause, it is a lost cause...unless we stabilise human numbers.
Thomas Malthus

India was the first country in the world to launch a National Family Planning Programme in 1952 with the objective of reducing the birth rate and controlling population. Family planning has been defined as 'a way of thinking and living that is adopted voluntarily upon the basis of knowledge, attitudes and responsible decisions by individuals and couples in order to promote the health and welfare of the family group and thus contribute effectively to the social development of the country'.

Adoption of contraception and preventing unwanted births has a positive influence on the health of the mother and children, reduces birth rates and controls population. The current status of these achievements is shown below (National Population Policy 2000).

Population	1 billion (100 crore)
Birth rate	26.4 per 1000 live births
Couple protection rate	44%
Infant mortality rate	72 per 1000 live births
Maternal mortality rate	437 per 1,00,000 live births

Factors like education, socioeconomic status, age, parity, and religion influence the clients' behaviour. The doctor should also consider the possibility of certain medical and gynecological disorders which if present, will govern the choice of contraceptives. While there is a wide range of contraceptives available for the woman, the choice is very limited for the men. The aim of the healthcare provider should be to help the client choose a contraceptive that is most acceptable to the couple. This is best done through the process of counselling as against the currently employed 'paternalistic' advice.

Objectives

At the end of this chapter, the reader should be able to

- ☐ List the different methods of contraception.
- ☐ Appreciate the efficacy of various contraceptives.
- ☐ Enumerate their side effects and complications.
- ☐ Appreciate factors that influence the acceptance of contraception.
- ☐ Counsel a client regarding contraception.
- ☐ Help the clients to choose an appropriate contraception.
- ☐ Prescribe contraceptives appropriately.

CLINICAL SCENARIO

A 23-year-old woman, a second para, seeks contraceptive advice.

HISTORY

It is important to elicit information regarding factors that influence the contraceptive advice.

1. ***Age***—The client is 23 years old; she can therefore use any of the contraceptives available in the market. Combination oral contraceptives (COC) pills are best suited for teenagers as their efficacy is good and because this age group is unlikely to have any medical disorders. If their sexual activity is unplanned, the choice is between the use of emergency contraception or use of condom by the male partner. Intrauterine contraceptive devices (IUCD) are not usually advised in nulliparous women since they cause severe cramps and there is also the risk of pelvic infection, which may subsequently lead to infertility. Recently married couples, similarly should be advised to take combination OC pills.

   In contraceptive terminology, middle age is considered as 35 years. In these women, OC pills should be given with caution as they may be suffering from medical disorders. Tubectomy should not be performed before 21 years and after 45 years of age according to the National Family Planning guidelines.

2. ***Parity*** per se does not preclude the use of any contraceptive, though an IUCD is preferably avoided in nullipara. The under five mortality rate is quite high in India. Therefore one should not advocate permanent methods like tubectomy or vasectomy, if the couple has only one child below the age of five years or a second child below 1 year, although the procedures for reversal are associated with an acceptable success rate, particularly in the case of tubectomy.

Currently, a number of women opt for tubectomy if they have two or more living children. Tubectomy can be performed during the puerperium, along with medical termination of pregnancy or in the postmenstrual phase. However, a client may continue using an IUCD, if she wishes, provided she gets it changed every 3–5 years. The other option is vasectomy particularly if the woman has some medical disorders and administration of anesthetic is associated with a risk.

3. ***Lactation*** will not protect a woman unless her baby is less than six months old, menstruation has not resumed and she is exclusively breast-feeding. COC pills are contraindicated as the quality and quantity of breast milk may be altered. Non-hormonal methods or injectables may be more suitable for women who are lactating.

4. It is essential to record the client's ***menstrual history*** carefully. Particular attention should be paid to irregular cycles, intermenstrual bleeding/contact bleeding and excessive bleeding. COC pills are useful in women with polymenorrhea and menorrhagia due to dysfunctional uterine bleeding.

Make a note of when the client had her last menstrual period (LMP). This information has a bearing on the administration of some contraceptives. For example, an IUCD is inserted in the postmenstrual phase, or the client should start taking OC pills from the second or the fifth day of the menstrual cycle.

5. One must enquire carefully to find out if the client seeking contraception has any ***medical disorders***.

   ❧ Oral contraceptives are contraindicated in women suffering from cardiovascular diseases, hepatic disorders and in diabetes mellitus with vascular complications. In case of hypertension, if the blood pressure is less than 160/100, COC pills containing 20 µg of estrogen may be prescribed. Injectable or subdermal implants containing medroxy progesterone acetate are acceptable alternatives.

   ❧ Rheumatic heart disease continues to be fairly common in India. For these clients, IUCD insertion with the threads cut very short to reduce the risk of infection, or tubectomy operation performed with adequate precautionary measures, is suitable. Infective endocarditis prophylaxis must be instituted prior to these procedures.

✤ COC pills are contraindicated if there is history of thromboembolic phenomena. Either IUCD or a combined use of condom and intravaginal spermicidal gel are good options.

✤ If a client is on treatment for tuberculosis, the efficacy of COC pills is reduced because of drug interaction between estrogen and rifampicin; so also in case of anti-convulsant therapy. She may be advised to use some other method.

6. *Education and socioeconomic status* influences the choice of contraceptives. An educated client is in a better position to use COC pills which have to be taken every day. She will understand the need to use a backup method if she forgets to take the pills. In the case of injectable/implant contraceptives amenorrhea and irregular bleeding are common side effects. Besides, most of the hormonal contraceptives are expensive, making it more suitable for the affluent except for the ones which are socially marketed.

Similarly, barrier methods like the vaginal diaphragm are better accepted by the educated because they can understand better the procedure of insertion and method of cleaning. The male condom is gaining acceptance among clients from different strata in the society, especially for the prevention of AIDS.

For clients from the poorer socioeconomic strata, IUCD has proved to be the best method for spacing as it requires only two visits to the healthcare facility, one for the insertion and one for follow up.

7. Clients belonging to certain *religions* refuse to use contraceptives and prefer natural methods, which are based on avoiding sexual intercourse in the periovulatory period. In Billing's method, the female client is asked to maintain a menstrual calendar and identify the 'wet feeling' in the vulva due to an increased amount of cervical mucus indicative of impending ovulation. Both the partners must understand that the failure rate of this method is quite high.

8. *Gender bias*—Very often, the responsibility of adopting contraception rests with the female partner. This is particularly true in India. Many men mistakenly believe that vasectomy is associated with loss of libido and an increased risk of prostatic cancer and myocardial infarction. The family may also prevent them from undergoing vasectomy, as they are the bread winners. There is certainly a need to allay these apprehensions and explain to them that vasectomy is a safer, simpler

and less expensive operation than tubectomy.

PHYSICAL EXAMINATION

This examination is performed with a view to detect pallor, hypertension, abnormalities in the breasts and any lesion in the cardiovascular and respiratory systems. Varicose veins must be looked for.

Abdominal examination

One should look for presence of any mass such as fibroids/ovarian tumours; liver and spleen must be palpated.

Vaginal speculum examination

One must check for infections which should be treated before inserting an IUCD. Any contraception is contraindicated in the presence of neoplastic lesion in the cervix or the vagina. **A Pap smear should be taken at this stage.** A **bimanual vaginal examination** is useful in confirming the diagnosis of fibroid or ovarian tumour and tubo-ovarian masses. In all these cases, contraceptives are contraindicated.

Further investigations should be conducted, if warranted by the history and physical findings.

No contraceptive should be prescribed for the woman in the presence of unexplained vaginal bleeding.

INVESTIGATIONS

An estimation of hemoglobin and urinalysis should be performed for all clients. Other tests like liver function tests, blood sugar, serum lipids, ultrasonography, and endometrial biopsy should be done when indicated.

Table 36.1 gives guidelines about contraceptive choices in common clinical situations.

NON-CONTRACEPTIVE BENEFITS OF CONTRACEPTION

Some contraceptives have added benefits. For example, OC pills regularise menstrual cycle, reduce the amount of bleeding and hence control anemia; logically, OC pills reduce the risk of ovarian cancer and endometrial cancer.

Barrier contraceptives, especially condoms, protect the clients against sexually transmitted diseases and HIV infection.

Table 36.1 Guidelines for contraceptive choices in common clinical situations

	Situation	Suitable method
I.	Newly married Adolescents Nullipara	Combined oral contraceptive (Avoid IUCD)
II.	Recently delivered	IUCD after 6 weeks (Avoid combined pills)
III.	Multipara	Vasectomy/tubectomy a) If there are ≥ 2 children b) If the second child is at least one year old
IV.	Women > 35 years	a) IUCD b) Injectable progestogens c) Progestogen only pills; two tablets of levonorgestrel 750 µg 12 hours apart; the first one within 72 hours of coitus and a second tablet after 12 hours not later than 16 hours
V.	Commercial sex workers (multiple sexual partners) History of pelvic infection/ectopic pregnancy	Oral pill + condom (male or female) (Avoid IUCD)
VI.	Rheumatic heart disease	Vasectomy/tubectomy IUCD with short tail Injectable progestogens Barrier + spemicides
VII.	Diabetics	Injectable progestogens Barrier + spermicides
VIII.	Emergency contraceptive	a) Two tablets of levonorgestrel 750 µg 12 hours apart; the first one within 72 hours of coitus and a second tablet after 12 hours not later than 16 hours b) IUCD within 5 days of coitus c) Oral pills 2 tablets twice at 12 hours interval not later than 72 hours after coitus

COUNSELLING

Counselling is a process where a balanced presentation is made to clients, of the available information regarding contraceptives, their benefits, side effects and above all the chances of failure of contraceptives (Table 36.2). Clients should be encouraged to clarify their queries so that they can choose a method of contraception most acceptable to them. Counselling consists of six steps that can be easily remembered by the acronym GATHER.

G *Greet* clients. Give them full respect and attention. Assure privacy and confidentiality.

A *Ask* about their family planning and reproductive health experiences, their wishes and concerns about family planning.

T *Tell* clients about choices. Focus on methods that interest the client and also briefly mention other available methods.

H *Help* clients make their own choice. Encourage them to express opinions and ask questions and clear all their doubts. Consider medical eligibility criteria for the method chosen.

E *Explain* fully how to use the chosen method. Check that the clients understand fully how to use the method.

R *Return* visits should be encouraged. Let them come back for further advice or for more supplies at any time.

Once the process of counselling has been completed and the client has opted for a contraceptive method, informed consent must be taken. The Ministry of Health and Family Welfare in India has prepared standard consent forms for tubectomy/vasectomy to be used in all the government institutions. Any consent form should contain:

❖ the side effects/risks of the procedure
❖ the awareness of chances of failure
❖ the client's signature and her/his name below the signature

One of the reasons for clients discontinuing contraceptives is that they are not told about the possible side effects. The client must be made to understand that there is no contraceptive which is **ideal** (safe, cheap, easy to use and effective). The occurrence of minor side effects often takes them by surprise, for example, slightly increased bleeding or pain during one or two cycles with IUCD. If the client is made to understand that these side effects are **less risky than the risk of an unwanted pregnancy and termination** and if they are mentally prepared and are assured that these minor side effects are temporary and can be managed, continuation rates of contraceptive use is found to be better.

Table 36.2 Types of contraceptives and failure rates

Contraceptive	Failure rate (HWY) (per hundred women years)
a) Conventional	
Condom (male)	5–15
Vaginal diaphragm	2–5
Spermicides	11–18
b) Hormonal	
Combined oral contraceptive pills	0.3
Injectable hormones (DMPA, NET–EN)	1
Norplant	0.6–0.8
c) Surgical	
Female sterilisation (Pomeroy method)	0.1–0.3
Laparoscopic sterilisation	0.2–1.3
Vasectomy	0.1–0.2
d) Others	
Safe period	25–35
Cervical mucus method	3
Lactational amenorrhea	5–10
Withdrawal method	6.7

The client signs accepting that the above facts have been explained to her/him in a language which she/he understands. **Obtaining an informed consent and maintaining proper records about the procedure involved are absolutely mandatory.**

Key points

1. A wide variety of contraceptives is available in India.
2. There is a need to emphasise spacing methods; currently, IUCD is the most accepted spacing method.
3. Failure rates are highest for the 'safe period' method. This point should be made clear to the client. The client must be made aware of failure rates of other methods too.
4. Tubectomy and vasectomy are not 100 per cent reversible and require a relatively major surgery for reversal.
5. OC pills protect women against ovarian and endometrial cancer. Condoms protect the partners against sexually transmitted diseases.
6. The burden of fertility and its control falls on the female partner. Efforts should be made to improve male participation. Vasectomy is simpler and safer than tubectomy.
7. Counselling is essential for effective implementation of the family planning programme.
8. Informed consent must be obtained and accurate records maintained.

CHAPTER 37

Strategies for skill learning

ASHA OUMACHIGUI

The skill of doing, comes of doing.
Ralph Waldo Emerson

Obstetrics and gynecology is one of the specialties where students are expected to actually perform and learn. According to the Medical Council of India (MCI) regulations (1997), they are to spend not less than one month as 'resident pupil' in a maternity ward of a general hospital. During this period, the students are supposed to conduct at least 10 cases of labour under supervision and assist in 10 other cases. The reference is to development of **'skills'** to conduct a delivery. This chapter deals with the meaning and types of skills, and what efforts the teachers should make to ensure that the students learn the skills that are considered essential. Therefore, the focus should be more on **what the student should be able to do** rather than on **what the student knows** so that medical graduates are competent to perform in actual practice.

Objectives

At the end of this chapter, the reader should be able to

- ❏ Define skill.
- ❏ Classify skills.
- ❏ Enumerate the steps in skill learning.
- ❏ Enumerate the factors that affect skill learning.
- ❏ Plan strategies for skill learning.
- ❏ Appreciate the fact that skill learning is essential for rendering effective reproductive and child health services.

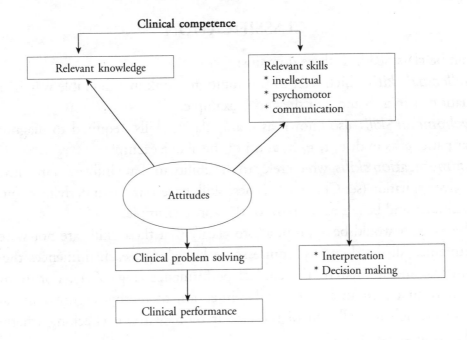

Fig. 37.1 Chart showing the influence of attitude on skill learning and clinical performance

Before proceeding further, it is important to clarify what is meant by a skill.
Definition—A skill is an ability to act appropriately in response to a situation.
It represents the results of employment of a specific combination of abilities applied to
a given task. For example, management of PPH requires:

a. recognition of excessive vaginal bleeding after delivery as harmful to the patient
b. recalling that in most cases atony is the cause of PPH
c. anticipating hypovolemic shock
d. starting an IV line with an 18 G cannula
e. collecting blood for crossmatching
f. administering methyl ergometrine
g. infusing Ringer lactate till blood is available
h. examining to ascertain uterine contraction
i. allaying the patient's apprehension and
j. monitoring her closely

CLASSIFICATION

Skills can be classified into three domains:

* *Intellectual skills* which refer to the ability to think in a desirable way in a given situation as in **a, b** and **c** of the above example.
* *Psychomotor skills* also known as manipulative skills, required to diagnose and treat patients as in **d, e, f, g, h,** and **j** of the above example.
* *Communication skills*, which refer to the ability to share information with others in a given situation (see Chapter 1). These skills have a strong underlying component of attitudes and beliefs as in step **i** of the above example.

At this stage it would be appropriate to clarify that these skills are not watertight compartments. All the domains require some knowledge, each influences the other two domains, and ultimately, the clinical performance (Fig. 37.1). For example, a student may first give an intramuscular injection of methyl ergometrine and be indifferent enough to walk out of the labour room without checking whether the uterus has contracted or not.

BASIC STEPS OF SKILL LEARNING

Skill learning is an active process and needs repeated practice.

The preliminary steps are as represented in the following learning sequence:

* Hearing and/or reading the description of the skill
* Observing a demonstration of the skill
* Practice under supervision, and later on, independently

It is worthwhile to see how these steps can be applied to skills in the three domains.

i) *Intellectual skills*—The steps involved in problem solving, which is the basis of arriving at a diagnosis and instituting treatment, are below:

* Learning basic facts, concepts and principles; for example, definition of PPH, cause of PPH and pharmacology of oxytocic drugs
* Solving a problem under guidance, managing PPH under supervision at every step
* Solving a problem with hints/clues—guided practice
* Solving a problem independently

ii) ***Psychomotor skills***—Learning these involves the following sequence:
   ❖ Listening or reading up about the component of skills especially elements of relevant procedure such as starting an IV line
   ❖ Watching a demonstration of the skills when the teacher points out each step
   ❖ Practising the skill under supervision
   ❖ Practising the skill independently

iii) ***Communication skills***—Learning these involves the following sequence:
   ❖ Listening to narratives, orations or inspiring anecdotes; mark the emotional component here. Watching the teacher motivating a relative to donate blood; watching and participating in role play, for example acting out a situation, such as, what happens when a pregnant mother is informed by the doctor that she is HIV positive.
   ❖ Practising under guidance
   ❖ Practising independently

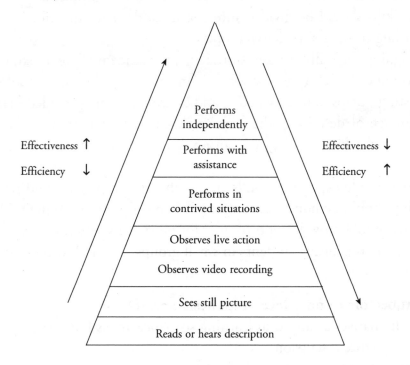

Fig. 37.2 Cone of experience

Factors affecting skill learning

a. Effectiveness is the quality of a learning experience which helps in achieving a **learning objective**. It depends on the realistic nature of the learning experience. The closer a learning experience is to reality, the more effective it is; for example watching *an actual case of PPH* is more effective than watching a video recording.

b. Effectiveness of skill learning is directly proportional to the degree of *active participation*. Efficiency is the quality of a learning experience which helps in achieving learning objective with minimum expenditure of time and other resources.

Various learning experiences could be diagramatically represented on a cone called the 'cone of experience' (Fig. 37.2). Effectiveness and efficiency have an inverse relation. As one goes up the cone, effectiveness increases and efficiency tends to decrease.

Role of the teacher in skill learning

❖ In the first place, the teacher must be convinced that the students should acquire predetermined skills. It is useful for the teacher to form a list of skills which the student must learn with reference to a particular clinical problem.

❖ Next, the skills should be divided into the three domains described earlier, and also according to their simplicity/complexity.

❖ While assigning the skill learning to students, the academic level of students must be kept in mind. For example, importance must be placed on methodology in the initial postings. Steps in history taking and examination are provided as handouts. The advantage of describing the steps is that it can be used at the end of the postings as a checklist to carry out an objective structured clinical examination (OSCE).

❖ The teacher should explain the skills and its theory components and relevance.

❖ The teacher should demonstrate the correct steps of performing the skill.

❖ The teacher should provide opportunities for practice by selecting cases, obtaining simulators, and organising students in small groups. The following is an example of a skill to be learnt.

Performing tubectomy under local anesthesia and sedation

Instructional alternatives arranged in learning sequence are as follows:

❖ Attending a lecture discussion

❖ Observing video demonstration of an operation

❖ Observing an operation on a client

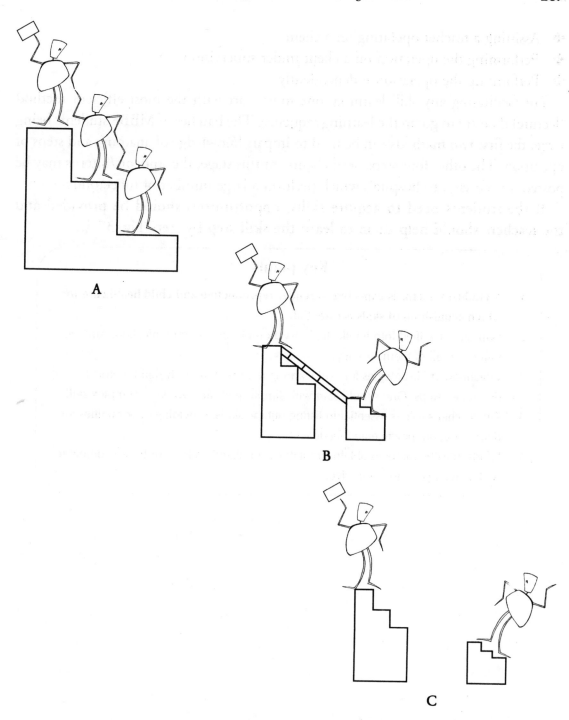

Fig. 37.3 Helping students learn; A: Desirable; B: Can be improved upon; C: Undesirable

❖ Assisting a teacher operating on a client
❖ Performing the operation on a client under supervision
❖ Performing the operation independently

For facilitating any skill learning, one must start with the most efficient method (lecture) then try to go up the learning sequence. The batches of MBBS students being large, the first two methods can be used to impart knowledge of anatomy and steps of operation. The other four steps need clients. At this stage, the students/interns may be posted if necessary, to hospitals which perform a large number of tubectomies.

If the students need to acquire skills, opportunities should be provided and the teachers should help them to learn the skill step by step (Fig. 37.3).

Key points

1. **A graduate doctor is expected to render reproductive and child healthcare for which acquisition of skills is essential.**

2. Skills are classified into intellectual, psychomotor and communication. Attitude influences all of them strongly.

3. Organisation of strategies for skill learning requires that each skill be broken down into steps. One should start with simple skills and go on to complex skills.

4. The teacher's role is essential in listing out the skills, providing opportunities for demonstration, practice and feedback.

5. Efforts must be made to obtain simulators, simulated patients or to use computers (virtual reality) as an alternative.

Bibliography

1. **Arias F** 1993. *Practical Guide to High Risk Pregnancy and Delivery.* 2nd ed, Mosby Year Book St. Louis.
2. **Arulkumaran S,** Ratnam S S and Bhasker Rao K 1996. *The Management of Labour.* Orient Longman, Chennai.
3. **Avery G B,** Fletcher M A and Mac Donald M G 1999. *Neonatology: Pathophysiology and Management of the Newborn.* W.B. Saunders, Philadelphia.
4. **Berek S,** Adashi E Y and Hillard P A 1996. *Novak's Gynaecology.* 12th ed, Williams and Wilkins, Baltimore.
5. **Bhakoo O N** 1980. Neonatal bacterial infection at Chandigarh – a decade of experience. *Ind J Pediatr* 47: 419.
6. **Bhat B V,** Pandey K K, Raghavan M 1994. Bacteriological profile of blood culture isolation from neonates. *Ind J Mat Child Health* 5: 114.
7. **Bhatt R V** 1996. A Report on Maternal Mortality in India: Project Sponsored by the WHO and the Ministry of Health and Family Welfare, New Delhi.
8. **Bloom R S,** Cropley C R N, and Charles R D. *Textbook of Neonatal Resuscitation.* American Heart Association.
9. **Brockington I** 1982. *Motherhood and Mental Illness.* Grune and Stratton, New York.
10. **Buckshee K,** Patwardhan V B and Soonawala R P 1996. *Principles and Practice of Obstetrics and Gynecology for Postgraduates.* Jaypee Brothers Medical Publishers, New Delhi.
11. **Carp H J A,** Toder V, Mashiac H S, et al 1990. Recurrent miscarriage: a review of current concepts, immune mechanisms and results of treatment. *Obstet Gynecol* 45: 657.
12. **Chaudhuri S K** 1998. *Practice of Fertility Control.* 4th ed, B.I. Churchill Livingstone, New Delhi.
13. **Clain A** 1998. *Hamilton Bailey's Demonstration of Physical Signs in Clinical Surgery.* 18th ed, John Wright and ELBS, Bristol.
14. **Cloherty J P** and Stark A R 1987. *Manual of Neonatal Care.* 2th ed, Medical Service International, Tokyo.
15. **Cox J L,** Holden J N and Sagovski R 1987. Detection of postnatal depression. Development of the 10 item Edinburgh Postnatal Depression Scale. *Br J Psych* 150: 782.
16. **Cunningham F G,** MacDonald P C and Gant N F et al 2001. *Williams' Obstetrics.* 21st ed, Prentice Hall International, New Jeresy.

17. **Daftary S N** and Chakravarty S 1998. *Holland and Brews' Manual of Obstetrics.* 16th ed, B.I. Churchill Livingstone, New Delhi.

18. **Das S** 1996. *A Manual on Clinical Surgery including Special Investigations and Differential Diagnosis.* 4th ed, S. Das, Calcutta.

19. **Davidson J** and Robertson E 1985. A follow up study of post partum illness. *Acta Psych Scand* 71: 45.

20. **De Swiet M** 1995. *Medical Disorders in Obstetric Practice.* 3rd ed, Blackwell Science, Edinburgh.

21. **DeCherney A H** and Pernoll M L 1994. *Current Obstetric and Gynecologic Diagnosis and Treatment.* 8th ed, Appleton and Lange, Norwalk.

22. **Donald I** 1979. *Practical Obstetric Problems.* 5th ed, Lloyd-Luke (Medical Books) London.

23. **Gregoire A J,** Kumar R, Everitt B et al 1996. Transdermal Oestrogen for Treatment of Severe Postpartum Depression. *Lancet* 347: 930.

24. **Haagensen C D** 1986. *Diseases of the Breast.* 3rd ed, W.B. Saunders, Philadelphia.

25. **Hant D M** and Norman J 2000. *Gynecology Illustrated.* Churchill Livingstone, London.

26. **Hatcher R A,** Rinehast W, Blackburn R, et al 1997. *The Essentials of Contraceptive Technology: A Handbook for Clinical Staff.* Johns Hopkins Population Information Programme, Baltimore.

27. **Hendrick V,** Altshuler L L and Suri R 1998. Hormonal changes in the postpartum and implications for postpartum depression. *Psychosomatics* 39: 93.

28. **Interpersonal Communication Skills: Training Manual** 1995. United Nations Population Fund. UNFPA Country Support Team. Office for South and West Asia, Kathmandu.

29. **Kennedy H** and Grath 1989. Maternity Blues. Detection and Measurement by Questionnaire. *Br J Psych* 155: 356.

30. **Lawson J B** and Stewart D B 1967. *Obstetrics and Gynaecology in the Tropics.* English Language Book Society, London.

31. **Llewellyn-Jones D** 1994. *Fundamentals of Obstetrics and Gynaecology.* 6th ed, Mosby Year Book, Sydney.

32. **Lumley J S P** 1997. *Hamilton Bailey's Physical Signs.* 18th ed, Butterworth–Heinemann, Oxford.

33. **Maberry M C,** Gilstrap L C, Bawdon R E, et al 1991. Anaerobic coverage for intra amniotic infection: maternal and perinatal impact. *Am J Perinatol* 8: 338.

34. **Medical Council of India** 1997. Regulations on Graduate Medical Education Medical Council of India, New Delhi.

35. **Mondal G P,** Raghavan M, Bhat B V et al 1991. Neonatal septicemia among inborn and outborn babies in a referral hospital. *Ind J Pediatr* 58: 529.

36. **Monif G R G** 1991. Intrapartum bacteriuria and postpartum endometritis. *Obstet Gynecol* 78: 248.

37. **National Population Policy 2000.** Department of Family Welfare, Ministry of Health and Family Welfare, Government of India, New Delhi.

38. **Nelson W E,** Beharman R E, Kleigman R H et al 1996. *Nelson's Textbook of Paediatrics.* 15th ed, W.B. Saunders, Philadelphia.

39. **Oumachigui A** and Bupathy A 1991. A competency based curriculum for primary prevention of obstructed labour. *Ind J Obstet Gynecol* 40: 1991.

40. **Padubidri V** and Daftary S N 1999. *Shaw's Textbook of Gynecology.* 12th ed, B.I. Churchill Livingstone, New Delhi.

41. **Palaniappan B** (Ed) 1997. *Mudaliar and Menon's Clinical Obstetrics.* 9th ed, Orient Longman, Chennai.

42. **Park K** 1998. *Park's Textbook of Preventive and Social Medicine.* 16th ed, Banarasi Das Bhanot Publishers, Jabalpur.

43. **Robertson N R C** 1988. *Textbook of Neonatology.* 1st ed, Churchill Livingstone, London.

44. **Rudolph A M** 1991. *Rudolph's Pediatrics.* 17th ed, Appleton and Lange, California.

45. **Seaward P G,** Hannah M E, Mysh T L et al 1997. International multicentre term prelabour rupture of membrane study: evaluation of predictors of clinical chorioamniotis and fever in patients with prelabour rupture of membranes. *Am J Obstet Gynecol* 177: 1024.

46. **Seshadri S** 1997. Nutritional anaemia in south Asia – a regional profile. UNICEF Regional Office for South Asia, New Delhi.

47. **Sethuraman K R** and Santhosh Kumar 1996. Implementing Innovation in Clinical Skills Training. (Proceedings of a Workshop – Supported by the WHO Grant-in-Aid) National Teacher Training Centre, Jawaharlal Institute of Postgraduate Medical Education and Research, Pondicherry.

48. **Speroff L,** Mitchell C, Glass R H al et 1998. *Clinical Gynaecologic Endocrinology and Infertility.* 5th ed, Williams and Wilkins, Philadelphia.

49. **Stanford J P,** David A, Tyrrell et al 1993. *Kass Handbook of Infectious Disease: Obstetric and Perinatal Infection.* Mosby Year Book, St. Louis.

50. **Studd J** 1995, 1998. *Progress in Obstetrics and Gynaecology,* Volumes 11 and 13, B.I. Churchill Livingstone, London.

52. **Swash M** 1997. *Hutchison's Clinical Methods.* 20th ed, Bailliere Tindall, London.

53. **Task Force Study** 1992. Evaluation of the nutritional anaemia prophylaxis programme. Indian Council of Medical Research, New Delhi.

54. **Tindal V R** 1986. *Jeffcoate's Principles of Gynecology.* 5th ed, Butterworths, London.

55. **Turnbull A** and Chamberlain G 1999. *Obstetrics.* 6th ed, Churchill Livingstone, London.

56. **Whitfield C R** 1995. *Dewhurst's Textbook of Obstetrics and Gynaecology for Postgraduates.* 5th ed, Blackwell Science, Edinburgh.

Index